Jacobo Schifter, PhD
Johnny Madrigal, MSc

The Sexual Construction of Latino Youth
Implications for the Spread of HIV/AIDS

Pre-publication
REVIEWS,
COMMENTARIES,
EVALUATIONS . . .

"**O**ne of the few studies to have looked systematically at how young people really live their lives, the meanings that underpin their sexual practices, and the consequences of this as it relates to HIV/ AIDS. *The Sexual Construction of Latino Youth* illustrates graphically how religious, gender, and scientific discourses combine together (and are resisted) so as to influence young people's actions. While the focus is on Latin American youth, the analysis offered has wide relevance elsewhere. This book is a must for those who recognize the need to rethink our understandings of young people and their behavior in its rightful cultural context."

Peter Aggleton
Director, Thomas Coram Research Unit Institute of Education, University of London, England

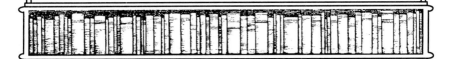

"**V**ery few times, if ever, has Latino youth sexuality been analyzed in such a comprehensive and illuminating way. The complex interaction of gender, class, religion, sexual orientation, and ethnicity—among other factors—is exposed here in all its richness.

This book is a must for teachers, social science researchers and students, health and HIV/AIDS educators and activists, parents, clergy members, and anyone interested in Latino cultures. It prompts the reader to reflect on how strongly religious and social ideologies shape our lives and, at the same time, how human beings always resist and find outlets to exert their freedom and reshape their lives, even in the least supporting environments. And finally, it shows with a sharp light how effective interventions in sexual health issues need to be conducted from a multilevel approach, including empowerment, awareness-raising techniques, socioeconomic changes, and political organization."

Alejandra Sardá, MA
Coordinator of Escrita en el Cuerpo,
Lesbian, Bisexual, and Different
Women's Archives and Library,
Woman's Secretariat,
International Lesbian
and Gay Association,
Buenos Aires, Argentina

The Sexual Construction of Latino Youth

Implications for the Spread of HIV/AIDS

THE HAWORTH HISPANIC/LATINO PRESS
Latin Sexuality
Jacobo Schifter, PhD, Senior Editor

Public Sex in a Latin Society by Jacobo Schifter

The Sexual Construction of Latino Youth: Implications for the Spread of HIV/AIDS by Jacobo Schifter and Johnny Madrigal

The Sexual Construction of Latino Youth
Implications for the Spread of HIV/AIDS

Jacobo Schifter, PhD
Johnny Madrigal, MSc

The Haworth Hispanic/Latino Press
An Imprint of The Haworth Press, Inc.
New York • London • Oxford

Published by

The Haworth Hispanic/Latino Press, an imprint of The Haworth Press, Inc., 10 Alice Street, Binghamton, NY 13904-1580

Cover design by Monica L. Seifert.

Cover photo © 1999 by Mark V. Lynch and Latent Images Photography. This photograph may not be copied, reproduced, or used in any manner whatsoever without prior written permission from: Mark V. Lynch, 6402 Evangeline Trail, Austin, TX 78727, USA, Phone (512) 250-2106, e-mail: mark@latentimages.com. Federal law provides penalties for copyright infringement. 1-800-944-4946. http://latentimages.com.

Library of Congress Cataloging-in-Publication Data

Schifter, Jacobo.
    The sexual construction of Latino youth : implications for the spread of HIV/AIDS / Jacobo Schifter, Johnny Madrigal.
        p.   cm.
    Includes bibliographical references and index.
    ISBN 0-7890-0884-X. — ISBN 0-7890-0885-8 (pbk.)
    1. Youth—Costa Rica—Sexual behavior. I. Madrigal Pana, Johnny. II. Title.
HQ27 .S257   2000
306.7'0835'097286—dc21   99-39463
                                                                                      CIP

CONTENTS

ABOUT THE AUTHORS

Jacobo Schifter, PhD, is the Regional Director of ILPES (the Latin American Health and Prevention Institute), an AIDS-prevention program financed by the Netherlands' government. One of the most prolific writers in Latin America, Dr. Schifter has written books on the Costa Rican civil war, U.S.-Costa Rican relations, and Costa Rican anti-Semitism before shifting his interests when AIDS started to affect the Central American region. He then established the first regional institute to fight the epidemic and created dozens of innovative programs, such as AIDS hotlines and AIDS-prevention workshops for Latin gays, prisoners, street children, Indians, male sex workers, and other minority groups. Dr. Schifter has also written several controversial books on AIDS, including *The Formation of a Counterculture: AIDS and Homosexuality in Costa Rica* (1989), *Men Who Love Men* (1992), *Eyes That Do Not See: Psychiatry and Homophobia* (1997), *Lila's House* (Haworth, 1998), *From Toads to Queens* (Haworth, 1999), and *Macho Love* (Haworth, 1999). These books have become best-sellers in the region and have also played a part in changing many Latin governments' discriminatory policies against people with AIDS.

Johnny Madrigal, MSc, is the Research Director of ILPES (the Latin American Health and Prevention Institute), an AIDS-prevention program financed by the Netherlands' government.

Foreword

I am delighted to be able to introduce this excellent book, and to provide a little of the background as to how the research described came about.

In 1992, when the Global Program on AIDS was in full swing at the World Health Organization headquarters in Geneva, I was invited to work as a consultant in the Social and Behavioral Studies (SSB) team for a few months. One of my tasks was to produce a review of what was then known regarding young people's sexual conduct across the world. What I found was that the majority of the studies tended to fall into three categories. The first relied on standard social survey methods and aimed to gain an overview of the prevalence of various behaviors, levels of knowledge, attitudes, and related factors; the WHO had sponsored some of these in developing countries, and other were funded by charitable bodies in developed countries. They were generally epidemiological and nontheoretical in nature.

The second group of studies—mainly in the United States—were based on well-established social and health psychology models, and explored, for example, the influence of various theoretical dimensions on contraceptive use, age at sexual debut, and other indices. The third group was social anthropological in nature, and tended to describe local patterns in restricted geographical regions.

While many of the studies reviewed were interesting and revealing, it was clear that there was a large gap in the coverage of the field. There was little in between the large scale surveys describing population-based data, and the smaller intensively designed contextual studies of specific areas and social groups. Furthermore, it was apparent that the social psychological theories used to frame the U.S. work—which had been found to be to some extent useful in some health domains—were not readily suitable for the study of the much more complex area of sexual conduct.

Our own work in the United Kingdom, as well as that of the Women's Risk and AIDS Project (WRAP), and some work in the

Netherlands, had, for the previous few years, been using qualitative methods to explore many aspects of young people's sexual conduct. The focus was very much on the ways in which the research participants spoke about the area, their own feelings, reactions, decisions, pressures, and other dynamic aspects. This approach to the work was based on a strong belief that successful interventions to reduce the threat of HIV and other unwanted outcomes of sexual activity could only be designed if they were based on a full understanding of the contexts in which sexual activity occurred.

The acting head of SSB at the time was Benoit Ferry, a French demographer who felt at home with data collected in large surveys. Nevertheless, he was persuaded by the review—and the insights gained from the fledgling qualitative work in some European countries—to make some tentative suggestions to the Steering Committee (chaired by Tom Coates) regarding the commissioning of some relatively groundbreaking research. I began work on a draft protocol which would form the basis of a series of studies in various countries to explore the very real social and cultural contexts in which young people commence and sustain their sexual lives.

Benoit Ferry moved on soon after this, and the new head of SSB—Peter Aggleton—took up the challenge with great enthusiasm. When I had to return to my post in the United Kingdom, Gary Dowsett (then at Macquarrie University, Sydney) was brought over to Geneva, and continued to develop the protocol. Bids were invited from researchers in many countries and, after careful review, seven studies were selected for funding; these were Cambodia, Cameroon, Chile, Costa Rica, Papua New Guinea, the Philippines, and Zimbabwe. The studies took place between 1993 and 1995. A summary of each of these studies and a brief overview of some of the recurrent cross-national themes was published in a special issue of *Critical Public Health* in December 1998 (Volume 8, Number 4), and UNAIDS has recently finalized a longer version.

This book derives from the studies in Costa Rica. In my view, Jacobo Schifter and Johnny Madrigal have more than repaid the faith that the early GPA staff and committee had in the new approach; indeed, they have gone considerably further than any of us would have hoped. By such close examination of the discourses and the contradictions around young people's sexuality, they have provided a model of how valuable these methodological and theoretical approaches can be. The detailed coverage of all aspects of the research process ensures that the book will not only be of immense relevance and interest to those working in Latin America, but will also be a valuable resource for those working in the field of sexual conduct in other countries and regions as well.

Roger Ingham, PhD
Director, Center for Sexual Health Research
University of Southampton, U.K.

Acknowledgments

This study would never have been completed without the generous support of many individuals and organizations. First and foremost, we would like to express our gratitude to Peter Aggleton, Chief of the Social and Behavioral Studies and Support Unit of the World Health Organization's former Global Programme on AIDS. Not only did he provide us with invaluable technical advice, but he was also instrumental in securing WHO funding on our behalf.

We would also like to thank Dr. Ellyn Kaschak of the State University of San Jose, California, and Dr. Sara Sharratt of the University of California in Sonoma; both were of great help to our team of researchers and field workers. Moreover, Dr. Sharratt also assisted in preparing the interview guide and in training interviewers.

We must also acknowledge the tireless support provided by a number of ILPES staff members. Administrative director Rodrigo Vargas coordinated all logistical aspects of project implementation, as well as engaging in the transcription and preparation of data for analysis. Rolando Guevara, meanwhile, developed the database that was subsequently used to organize and analyze the research findings.

In similar fashion, special mention must be made of all those who were involved in the project as interviewers and transcribers. Among the former group are Abelardo Araya, Kattia Castellón, Jenny Castro, Kattia Chinchilla, Larissa Fallas, Glenn Fonseca, Tatiana Fonseca, Tamara Fuster, Carmen Gutiérrez, Allan Guzmán, Marla Hernández, Patricia Jones, Carmen León, Kattia López, Erick Quesada, César Rodríguez, Indira Rodríguez, Fresia Romero, Edgar Salgado, Vanessa Smith, Viria Solís, and Luis Villalta.

Transcribers included Víctor Calderón, Shirley Garbanzo, Marielos Gómez, Maritza Gómez, Carmen Gutiérrez, Grettel Gutiérrez, Guiselle Gutiérrez, Ester Jara, Natasha Jiménez, Mayela La Touche, Ana Yancy Madrigal, Hanny Martínez, Maureen Medrano, Randall

Medrano, Marco Quirós, Indira Rodríguez, Vanessa Rojas, Maricela Rueda, Ana Lorena Sánchez, Emilia Sancho, Graciela Vásquez and Lucía Zamora.

Finally, we would like to thank the people of "Villa del Mar" and "Villa del Sol" for welcoming us into their respective communities, and the young people interviewed for their cooperation and insights. Needless to say, the support of these groups was crucial to the overall success of the project.

The contents of this work, including any errors or omissions, are the responsibility of the authors alone.

Chapter 1

General Overview

STUDY RATIONALE AND OBJECTIVES

Latin America has a significantly lower HIV-infection rate than Africa or Asia. The region has 8.4 percent of the world's population, 5.3 percent of them living with AIDS. The epidemic is affecting more males than females (81 percent males, 19 percent females), but the rise in heterosexual transmission is narrowing the male-female gap. In 1997, 1.3 million Latin Americans were infected with HIV, with 232,523 new reported cases occurring within that year. More than 100,000 people had already died of AIDS and it is estimated that by the year 2000 the number will rise to 300,000. For 1999, 382,378 new AIDS cases are predicted. The epidemic is becoming the most common cause of death for people between twenty-five and forty years of age. Given the fact that a lapse as long as ten years occurs between infection and the onset of the disease, many were infected in their teens. In Honduras, with more than 50 percent of the Central American AIDS cases, 20 percent of the people living with AIDS are in the fifteen to twenty-four age range (Izazola, 1998).

The AIDS epidemic has served to highlight young people's vulnerability to sexually transmitted disease in Latin America. In those countries where KAP (knowledge, attitudes, and practice) studies have been carried out, it has been found that young people as a group are less informed on HIV prevention than adults and that many young people engage in practices which place them at high risk of contracting HIV (Izazola, 1998). In the face of this danger, in some countries the state has played a role in sex education, and its principal response has been to promote condom use through the media. However, its efforts in this regard have been effectively stymied by the leadership of the Roman Catholic Church, a potent force in Latin America, and one which deemed the condom campaign to be immoral.

Given this context, one of the purposes of the present work is (1) to analyze the sexual cultures of young people and their impact upon sexual practice in one country (particularly as this relates to the risk of HIV infection), and (2) to identify obstacles to sexual education and HIV prevention in a Latin context.

This study has additional important objectives. There is very little research on Latino sexual culture, particularly on youth. This lack of information hinders sex education and HIV-prevention efforts in all youth-related programs. There is considerable awareness that Latino culture is distinctive with regard to sexuality, yet at the same time little information on its special character and dynamics is available. The authors believe that Michel Foucault's theoretical insights on the construction of sexuality contribute to theoretical development in this field. He proposed to study cultural phenomena through the analysis of "discourses," which he defined as the tools needed to understand how individuals are all shaped by and at the same time empowered to change sexual culture.

This book will focus on young Latinos' "sexual discourses," the instrumental role they play in constructing sexual culture, and their particular impact on sex education and AIDS prevention. While Foucault centered his groundwork on discourses, he offered little help in operationalizing the concept and in exploring the origins, diversity of types, and rules by which they function. The present work will, therefore, attempt to expand the notions of what is understood by discourses.

Two different youth cultures in a Latin American country (Costa Rica) were selected to study the impact and typologies of discourses. If AIDS-prevention programs are to be effective, adequate account must be taken both of differences in sexual culture and the role of gender and class in producing such differences. Adopting a comparative approach, we sought initially to identify two communities—"Villa del Mar" and "Villa del Sol"—which differed widely in the socioeconomic background of their inhabitants, the quality of their social and physical infrastructure, their economic base and, last but not least, the sexual lives of their youth.

This work claims that in present-day Costa Rica, one may identify at least six major sexual discourses. The first three are hegemonic, and these we have labeled "religious," "gender-based," and "rational-scientific." Meanwhile, the last three are resistance discourses, and these may be termed "erotic," "romantic," and "feminist." As these discourses are not the exclusive domain of any single group—though admittedly some derive greater benefit from them than do others—contradictions and resistance are inevitable. Young people do not assimilate them mechanically, but rather transform them in ways that reflect their class and gender positioning. In this way, the sexual cultures of youth are subject to a constant process of (re)negotiation, with class and gender being but two of the variables at work in influencing the particular thrust of their evolution.

It is the authors' goal to identify aspects of sexual culture that are shared by a multiplicity of Latin American cultures. For this reason, we selected communities that were "typical" of the most developed Latin countries (Argentina, Chile, Uruguay) as well as of regions characterized by more poverty (Mexico, Central America, the Caribbean, the Andean countries). Nevertheless, it is also obvious to us that we cannot generalize our findings to the entire region. Latin America and the Hispanic communities are too diverse. We believe that the commonalities of religion, heritage, and language, among others, impact ideology and notions of gender, sexuality, identity, and expectations about the world. The findings can, hopefully, be relevant to young people living in Managua, New York, or Buenos Aires. It is our hope that this work will encourage other researchers to conduct similar studies in other countries and communities.

During the course of this study, "sexual culture" is used to refer to all sex-related discourses (messages) to which young people are exposed, their inherent contradictions, the forms of resistance they engender, and their role in the compartmentalization of feelings and thoughts. To highlight the discrepancies and contradictions inherent within these sexual cultures, we will carry out analyses in two communities that stand in sharp contrast to each other in terms of their socioeconomic characteristics: the first being marginal in orientation ("Villa del Mar"), the second overwhelmingly middle class

("Villa del Sol"). The names of the communities as well as all names of participants have been changed to ensure confidentiality.

It should be noted that our aim is merely to examine sexual discourses, discursive practices, and their relation to sexual culture, and *not* to undertake a comprehensive study of the myriad factors that may be related to sexual culture in one way or another. These we will address only indirectly, by exploring their role in changing sexual practices and discourses over time.

However, as important as the objectives outlined above may be, a final one remains crucial: the wish to explain how sexual cultures of Costa Rican youth relate to the spread of HIV/AIDS within this population.

STRUCTURE OF THE STUDY

This work is divided into thirteen chapters, with the first four being primarily introductory in nature. The first chapter summarizes the major findings, as well as outlining the study's rationale and organization. This in turn is followed by a contextualization of the research, consisting of a description of the participating communities, along with a discussion of sex education in Costa Rica and young people's sexual practices and awareness of HIV/AIDS. In the third chapter, we turn to questions of methodology, identifying specific objectives, providing detailed information on the study sample, research methods, principles underlying the preparation of the interview guide, and characteristics of the field staff hired to carry out the study. Meanwhile, Chapter 4 sets out the social constructionist framework that underpins our understanding of young people's sexual cultures. This chapter also includes a discussion of the characteristics of discourses, their place in sexual culture, and their impact on prevention. Particular stress is placed upon their origins, the means by which they are imposed, their contradictions, the forms of resistance they generate, and the effects they produce.

In Chapter 5, we explore the bases of hegemonic sexual discourses—religious, gender-based, and scientific—as they are internalized by the participants themselves. This in turn provides the necessary grounding for our discussion in Chapters 6, 7, and 8 of the ways in which class and gender affect their assimilation by young people. Then, in Chapter 9, we examine the various actors and coercive mechanisms at work in imposing and reinforcing the messages inherent within these discourses, while Chapter 10 encompasses an examination of their underlying contradictions, together with the gender- and class-specific coping strategies devised by young people to deal with them. Flowing from this discussion, Chapters 11 and 12 examine the patterns of formal and informal resistance engaged in by young people in the face of prevailing sexual discourses. Finally, in Chapter 13, we undertake an analysis of the range of obstacles sexual culture places in the way of effective prevention.

Chapter 2

Background

Costa Rica gained its independence in 1821, having been part of the Spanish empire for close to three centuries. At the time of initial contact with the European colonizers, the indigenous population of what is now Costa Rica did not exceed 25,000 (Thiel, 1977), making it one of the most sparsely populated regions of Central America.

During much of the colonial period, as in the rest of Latin America, Roman Catholicism enjoyed a monopoly over the minds and souls of the country's inhabitants, as it was the only religion tolerated by Costa Rica's Spanish rulers. At the economic level, the era of Spanish rule was characterized most notably by chronic poverty, with a lack of human resources and mineral wealth ensuring that there was little in the way of sustained growth. This placed the country in the same disadvantaged position as regions in Latin America without mineral wealth during the colonial period: Argentina, Chile, Venezuela, Colombia, Uruguay, and Central America with the exception of Honduras. Since economic growth developed around the mining industries and services oriented toward it, Spain built most of the infrastructure in the center of these industrial complexes. The rest of the region was undeveloped and neglected by the colonial authorities. Costa Rica attracted, therefore, little immigration throughout the three centuries of Spanish domination.

Although the country's peasant-based economy did establish sporadic links with the world market thanks to crops such as cocoa and tobacco (Roses, 1975; Acuña, 1978), it was not until the mid-nineteenth century, with the advent of widespread coffee cultivation, that Costa Rica was integrated into the global chain of commodity production and consumption on a more permanent basis (Hall, 1982; Cardoso and Pérez, 1977). The introduction in Latin America of export economies reversed the colonial pattern. The most backward and marginal economies were the first to make changes and adapt to the new demands. Since they lacked a bureaucratic and rigid economic system imposed by Spain and also supported by local elites, the poorer countries were able to dismantle tariffs and barriers earlier than those more deeply connected with Spain. Costa Rica for one was able to direct its economy toward coffee exports and foreign investments. The irony in Latin America was that those hitherto richer and more prosperous colonial economies (Mexico, Peru, Bolivia) would pay dearly for their colonial mineral booms. It also led them to numerous civil wars in their struggles to establish open economies. Costa Rica, on the other hand, had some of the fastest growth and development in Latin America during the nineteenth century. In the post–World War II period, government policies of import substitution galvanized the industrial sector while attracting large numbers of European immigrants, whose presence contributed in turn to an expansion of the country's ethnic and religious mix. At present, roughly 85 percent of Costa Rica's population calls itself Roman Catholic, while the rest self-identify with a range of Protestant and non-Christian religions.

The country today has a higher standard of living than many Latin American nations. Its per capita income in 1994 was $2,380. This makes it six times larger than Nicaragua's ($380), three times larger than Bolivia's ($770), and two times larger than the Dominican Republic's ($1,460). It is much smaller than Argentina's ($8,110), Uruguay's ($4,660), and Mexico's ($4,010) (*Almanaque Mundial*, 1999).

Hence, the country occupies a middle position in terms of per capita income but shows more development in social indexes. Costa Rica has one of the highest literacy percentage rates in Latin America (Cuba, 96.0; Costa Rica, 95.0; Brazil, 83.0; Bolivia, 83.0; and Guatemala, 55.0), one of the lowest children's mortality percent rates per 100,000 (Costa Rica, 13.0; Argentina, 24.0; Mexico, 34.0; Brazil, 47.0) and one of the highest life expectancy rates (Costa Rica: men—71.2, women—77.5; Cuba: men—71.9, women—77.5; Argentina: men—69.6, women—76.8; Brazil: men—56.7, women—66.8) (*Almanaque Mundial*, 1999).

Despite the undoubted contribution made by coffee to Costa Rica's economic growth, it also served to make the country extremely vulnerable to the boom and bust cycle of the world commodity market. The same can be said about the rest of the more open economies in Latin America. When commodity prices fell in the world market, unrest and political instability were unleashed. Economic recessions led to the famous military interventions during the 1900s in numerous Latin American republics such as Mexico and Peru. This was not true in Costa Rica, where the existence of an agricultural frontier zone until roughly the middle of the twentieth century contributed to the emergence of a large middle class and to the establishment of a democratic tradition that was interrupted only twice in this century. In 1948, following the second of these interruptions, Costa Rica's government abolished its armed forces.

In this way, the country was able to weave a social fabric in which polarization and anomie were never permitted to reach the levels seen in other parts of Latin America, where military dictatorship was the rule rather than the exception. The program of social reform first embarked upon by the government of Calderón Guardia in the 1940s, subsequently deepened and strengthened by Jose Figueres Ferrer's Social Democratic Party, laid the groundwork for a welfare state that put Costa Rica on par with First World countries in such areas as literacy and health. Notwithstanding the good achievements in health and social security, approximately one-third of Costa Rica's population lives below the poverty line (*Almanaque Mundial,* 1999). The country shares with the rest of the region problems of unemployment, urban decay, increasing crime rates, and drug-related problems.

SEX EDUCATION IN COSTA RICA

In Costa Rica, the Ministry of Public Education has attempted to promote sex education in schools through its "Population Education Project." However, despite receiving funding—and support—from UNESCO and the United Nations Fund for Population Activities, the ministry has been forced to contend with sustained opposition on the part of the Roman Catholic Church.

Church authorities argue that educational materials dealing with sex education contain a number of "moral irregularities," and thus have demanded not only that Church views on premarital sex, abortion, and birth control be included in the text, but that the materials themselves only be distributed by teachers of religion.

It is against this background that the Ministry of Public Education has made repeated attempts (since 1995) to produce an acceptable series of sex education manuals; yet even now one can scarcely claim that the ministry has a viable program in place. In short, not only is teachers' use of the manuals voluntary, but they are more a teaching aid than anything else. Even though they contain information that could potentially be useful to all educators, their structure is such that they are used primarily by teachers involved in orientation, home education, religious instruction, and science.

What this means in effect is that sex education is not compulsory in Costa Rican secondary schools, and that its presence in the curriculum depends upon individual schools and teachers. Of course, it does not help that arguments for and against sex education are highly polarized: while those in favor claim that it helps young people to sort out their problems, opponents believe that it serves principally to promote sexual activity. However, despite the latter claims, not only has research failed to establish a link between sex education and promiscuity or early onset of sexual activity (Madrigal and Schifter, 1990), but some have even argued that individuals who are not exposed to such instruction tend to undergo sexual initiation at a younger age, since they do not have the tools with which to make informed decisions (Madrigal and Schifter, 1990).

SEXUALITY AND YOUNG PEOPLE

Costa Rican sexual practices are not much different from those of the rest of Latin America. For a snapshot, consider the following data: 42 percent of births take place outside of marriage; 18 percent of unwed mothers are nineteen years of age or younger; almost half of pregnancies are unwanted; on average, 20 percent of marriages end in divorce; 35 percent of women have been subjected to physical or psychological abuse by their partners; 27 percent of university students report being victims of child sexual assault; and Costa Rican physicians perform roughly 5,000 abortions annually (Madrigal Pana, 1992; Cover, 1995; Brenes, 1994).

Needless to say, these figures are indicative of several key features of Costa Rican sexuality. Although it is not the purpose of the present study to undertake a definitive analysis of the matter, some context is crucial if the reader is to understand what follows. With this end in mind, we draw upon the findings from some of our earlier work in the area of sexuality.

In the first instance, with regard to young people's sources of information about sex, the *First National Survey on AIDS* shows quite clearly that, for almost half of young male respondents (fifteen to twenty-four years), the street was where most of their sex "education" took place. The situation is somewhat different for young women, with home (34 percent) and school (26 percent) being the principal sources of information for this group. Other sources of information for both males and females are books, magazines, and newspapers (7 percent for young men and 8 percent for young women), and the mass media (7 and 8 percent, respectively).

Despite the fact that no well-defined national policy on sex education is in place in Costa Rica, nonetheless a high proportion of young people are receiving some formal instruction on sex-related matters, including sexual organs (90 percent); childbirth, contraceptives, sexually transmitted diseases (STDs), menstruation and teenage pregnancy (70 percent), and HIV/AIDS (55 percent). Still, it is also clear that much of this instruction is traditional in its approach, with far greater emphasis on biology than psychology, and with little attempt made to speak directly to young people's concerns. Furthermore, because of dominant prejudices, there is a tendency to restrict STD instruction to young males and information about the menstrual cycle and pregnancy to young females.

As one might imagine, not only does this state of affairs serve to reinforce the already strongly sexist character of Costa Rican society, but it leaves youth ignorant of many of the basic elements of sexuality. For example, approximately 40 percent of young people do not know whether a girl is able to conceive after her first menstruation, and only 30 percent of respondents can accurately describe when in the menstrual cycle a woman is most likely to be fertile. It is obvious as well that large numbers of young people have fallen prey to sexual myths, with more than half of male and female respondents indicating that they believe masturbation to be harmful to their health and that vaccinations exist to prevent STD infection. Indeed, a surprising number of young people (44 percent of males and 29 percent of females) believe as well that there are special substances that may be used to make people fall madly in love. Of course, given the preponderance of these beliefs, it is not particularly surprising that many young men and women have their first sexual experience at an early age.

As for the question of whom young people talk to about sex, our research has shown that young men tend to confide mainly in their friends and classmates (64 percent), while only 7 percent discuss sexual issues with their parents. Young women by contrast tend to be more communicative, confiding in their mothers (29 percent), husbands (27 percent), and friends and classmates (23 percent). With regard to the level of intimacy in these discussions, one finds that it is generally low between fathers and their children (less than 35 percent for males and less than 20 percent for females), and highest between mothers and daughters, and between male respondents and their male friends or classmates.

RISK OF HIV INFECTION THROUGH SEXUAL CONTACT

Young people run the risk of HIV infection from the moment they become sexually active. For men, the average age of initiation is sixteen, with as many as 15 percent of boys having their first sexual experience at age fourteen or younger. Their first partner is usually a female acquaintance or girlfriend who is on average five years older than themselves. In the case of women, the average age of sexual initiation is nineteen, and usually takes place with a man who is five or six years older than they are, and who is generally their fiancé, boyfriend, or husband.

Only 13 percent of men and 18 percent of women report using some form of contraceptive during their first sexual encounter. As for condom use, the figures are even more discouraging: for both men and women, it is practically nil.

In terms of AIDS awareness, although one might argue that the population in general is well informed, youth in particular are not. For instance, almost half of young men do not realize that an individual can be HIV positive for more than five years without becoming ill, while fully one quarter of them do not know that AIDS is a life-threatening disease. Although some evidence suggests that young women are better informed than their male counterparts, it is clear that they suffer as well from a number of misconceptions. Most notably, almost three quarters of them do not know that mutual masturbation is a form of safe sex (as compared with 54 percent of young males), while 44 percent are ignorant of the fact that condom use lessens the likelihood of HIV infection (versus 12 percent for young men).

Of course, given the latter findings, one is not particularly surprised to learn that only 25 percent of sexually active males, and 16 percent of sexually active females, use condoms on a regular basis. The numbers become even more alarming when one turns to younger women, who are the least likely of all segments of the population to make regular use of condoms. Among youth who do engage in condom use, almost half report being dissatisfied with them, and indicate that they would prefer to use another form of family planning, were it available.

Taken together, the findings outlined above provide ample evidence in support of a proactive stance on AIDS prevention for young people, all the more so when one considers the fact that every month 27 percent of males and 17 percent of females between the ages of twenty and twenty-four take part in forms of sexual activity that place them at risk of HIV infection.

COMMUNITIES STUDIED

As already stated, the present study seeks to explore young people's sexual cultures through a comparative analysis of two communities with widely variant socioeconomic backgrounds. Having considered several options, we finally decided upon two candidates: Villa del Sol, in the center of the country, and Villa del Mar, on the seacoast.

Of course, in this regard it bears emphasis that the task of choosing appropriate communities for comparison and study was made that much more difficult by the lack of readily comparable data. In short, not only were we faced with the fact that no population or housing census has been carried out in Costa Rica since 1984, but, in many areas where useful data are available (such as birth and death registries and use of health care services), they are not available at the community level.

Villa del Sol extends over five square kilometers and its population was estimated to be 8,000 in 1993. Although no official figures are available that provide details of Villa del Mar's geography, we estimate its size to be roughly equivalent to that of Villa del Sol, while the most recent population estimates suggest that it had 14,200 inhabitants in 1994. According to health clinic staff in the two communities, youth (between ten and nineteen years of age) make up approximately 18 percent of Villa del Sol's population, and 24 percent of that of Villa del Mar.

As for the nature of the communities' economic base, official employment statistics indicate that 20 percent of Villa del Sol's working population was engaged in handicrafts and cottage industries; 19 percent in livestock farming; 17 percent in services; 10 percent in trade and sales; 9 percent in professional categories; 8 percent in the public sector or independent enterprises; and smaller percentages in a number of other sectors, including transportation, management, and administration. As these figures suggest, the town enjoys considerable diversity in economic activity, in sharp contrast to Villa del Mar. Although no quantitative data are available, it is clear that employment in Villa del Mar is for the most part concentrated in farming, animal husbandry, fishing, retail trade, tourism, and other maritime occupations. With regard to retail trade in particular, it is focused primarily upon the operation of taverns, grocery stores, and clothing boutiques.

While one is left to assume that unemployment is low in Villa del Sol (no official figures are available), owing to the diversity of its economic base, as many as 46 percent of Villa del Mar's able-bodied inhabitants are out of work. Needless to say, widespread joblessness does not lend itself to harmonious social relations.

How to explain these differences? Without wishing to suggest that this is the only factor at work, it is nonetheless clear that the two communities are characterized by widely disparate histories. Villa del Mar is less than forty years old, and was established through forced migration from overcrowded urban areas. By contrast, not only does Villa del Sol owe its growth to an earlier phase of (voluntary) immigration, but it has had much longer to develop its livestock farming, handicrafts, and industrial sectors.

In matters of health care, data provided by local clinic staff suggest that Villa del Mar's population is far more prone to illnesses related to poverty and unhygienic conditions than is the case for inhabitants of Villa del Sol. Needless to say, sewage and drainage systems in Villa del Mar provide insufficient capacity, particularly in the rainy season, and its health care resources are less than adequate given the needs of the population. These problems are aggravated by widespread drug addiction, alcoholism, and family violence in the town, which community leaders blame on chronically high rates of local unemployment.

Although no comparative data are available for literacy, primary school attendance is considered high for boys and girls in both communities. However, one assumes that attendance rates decrease in secondary and postsecondary school. As community leaders in Villa del Mar pointed out, a large proportion of teenagers drop out prematurely, owing to such problems as low family income, marital breakup, substance abuse, and prostitution.

Family characteristics also differ for each community. In Villa del Sol, the nuclear family remains the predominant model, with the majority of households characterized by the presence of both parents. This is not the case in Villa del Mar, where a social worker reported to us that three out of every four households were headed by women only. Furthermore, if one includes in this figure families in which the male parent is away for extended periods of time because of fishing or other out-of-town work commitments, the proportion of female single-parent families becomes even higher.

Also worthy of note in this regard is the wide disparity in religious practice. Despite the presence in the town of ten Protestant churches, it is obvious that Villa del Sol is a predominantly Roman Catholic community. Not only does it have twelve Catholic churches, but saints' feast days and high holidays invariably attract large crowds of devout worshipers. By contrast, in Villa del Mar the situation is quite different: Evangelical and Baptist churches predominate, while Roman Catholic ones are in the minority. While acknowledging that the number of churches is not necessarily the best predictor of the number of worshipers, one might nonetheless argue that Protestant fundamentalism is a considerably more potent force in Villa del Mar than in Villa del Sol.

Life in the Communities

Villa del Sol's rapid urban growth is all the more obvious when compared with the wide tracts of rural hinterland that surround it. Moreover, trade with this hinterland is clearly of great importance to the town's economy, as is attested by the large number of grocery stores (forty-eight), supermarkets, minimarkets, and suppliers (thirty), hardware stores, and woodworking and automobile repair shops (ninety-six), restaurants and fast-food eateries (forty-five), vegetable and fruit markets, flower shops, and tree nurseries (twenty-two), meat markets and farm accessory stores (seventeen), liquor merchants (fourteen), bakeries (ten), and beauty salons (sixteen), among others.

Not surprisingly, there is far less evidence of prosperity in Villa del Mar. Although there are some paved roads in the town, most are either gravel or dirt. Retail trade employs far fewer people, and contributes much less to the community's tax base: in stark contrast with Villa del Sol, there are only twenty-one grocery stores, two suppliers, three general stores, one automobile repair shop, six restaurants, and one meat market.

The respective wealth of each community can also be seen in the different types of housing construction. In Villa del Mar, most houses are made out of wood, and many are old and dilapidated. Where brick homes do exist, they were for the most part built with funds provided by the National Institute of Housing and Urban Development. However, even here the houses are in a poor state of repair, mostly because their occupants lack the necessary resources to maintain or enlarge them. Needless to say, this in turn has contributed to overcrowded conditions, with large families sharing very small quarters. As in other areas, the contrast with Villa del Sol is obvious. Here, most of the homes are of brick and in good condition, though admittedly there are some neighborhoods where housing stock is of lower quality.

Another significant difference between Villa del Sol and Villa del Mar shows in the attitude of community members. In the latter case, people are generally open and friendly. As one walks down the

street, one is often engaged in conversation or invited into someone's home. Villa del Mar's hot, humid climate ensures that people
dress in lightweight clothing, and bodies are exhibited with less
inhibition. Women tend to wear low-cut or halter tops with shorts
and sandals. Men often go shirtless, clothed only in Bermuda short-
s. Boys and girls are generally found barefoot, wearing identical
styles of clothing.

In Villa del Sol, people are far more reserved and tend to be
distrustful of strangers. They are loath to invite those they do not
know into their homes, and it is difficult as a stranger to make
friends or contacts. The style of dress is also more conservative;
bodies tend to be covered up, despite the warmth of the weather.
Most community members are practicing Roman Catholics, with
much of the town's social calendar revolving around the Church
and saints' feast days and, for young people in particular, around
the Boy Scouts or religious youth groups. In short, this is a community whose guiding principles are dictated by the Roman Catholic
Church, and whose people are reluctant to cross their parish priest
for fear of the social condemnation this may engender.

As for patterns of socialization in the two towns, one is immediately struck by the degree to which men and women in Villa del
Mar form segregated, single-sex groups, with the beach being one
of the few locales where there is widespread mixing among the
sexes. Aggression and teasing are common among groups of men.
As for women, they are seldom seen in large group settings, since,
as one participant explained, "It is very difficult to communicate
with girlfriends because they're usually trying to do you in, especially when there's a man involved." While there appears to be
more interaction between the sexes in Villa del Sol, with mixed
groups of males and females readily observable on the street, it is
nonetheless clear that they share many of the same communication
problems faced by young people in Villa del Mar.

The two communities are also characterized by considerable
variation in their leisure spaces. In Villa del Mar, the beach and city
plazas are by far the most popular places in which to congregate. On
weekends, young people tend to go to the beach during the day and
to one of the town's discotheques at night. In Villa del Sol, by
contrast, young people spend most of their leisure time in nearby

San José, though some can also be found in one of the town's two local dance clubs.

In matters of sex and reproduction, although little comparative data is readily available, birth registries show that young women under the age of twenty account for a significantly higher proportion of births in Villa del Mar (27 percent) than is the case in Villa del Sol (18 percent), thereby placing the community far above the national average for teenage pregnancies. At a purely anecdotal level, it should be noted that one often encounters pregnant adolescent girls on the streets of Villa del Mar, a sight that is comparatively rare in Villa del Sol. Of course, given these observations, one is not surprised to learn that early marriage (either de facto or de jure) due to pregnancy is commonplace in Villa del Mar, a finding confirmed by project ethnographers, and which stands in sharp contrast to Villa del Sol, where cohabitation by young people is relatively rare.

Sexual Contexts

As one might imagine, Villa del Sol and Villa del Mar offer their young people widely divergent possibilities in the sexual realm. In the case of Villa del Sol, its proximity to the San José metropolitan area, with a population of close to a million, ensures that its youth have no shortage of opportunities for fraternizing with prospective sexual partners, whether in bars, discos, brothels, athletic clubs, private parties, or movie theaters. It is clear that their own community also provides ample scope for socialization, with young people meeting each other at church functions, or in coffee houses, parks, and billiard halls. On Sunday evenings in particular, many young people can be found in the city square, where they mingle with their friends and seek out appropriate partners. However, it should be noted that the same does not apply to Villa del Sol's gays and lesbians, who tend to travel to San José for their leisure activities, rather than run the risk of being spotted by someone they know.

As one strolls around the town's main square in the evening, one is immediately struck by the number of young couples holding hands or kissing, while groups of adolescent boys and girls congregate in front of the church's main gate. Other popular hang-outs for young people are the town's many coffee houses (*sodas* in local parlance), which serve as fast-food eateries during the day, and social centers in the evening. Young couples come to chat with friends or each other, while unattached adolescents gather together at the larger tables.

As the evening progresses, couples make their way to the municipal park, which is poorly lit and hence ideal for those wishing to engage in sexual intercourse without being seen. Also popular in this regard is the dark area behind the church, where couples come to fondle one another and have sex.

While Villa del Mar is also close to a large urban center, the latter is considerably smaller than San José (it is roughly one-tenth its size), and hence characterized by significantly fewer social establishments. However, as one of Costa Rica's principal port cities, it does have more than its share of bars and brothels, which serves to reinforce its reputation as a sexual mecca for those living in nearby towns and villages.

Villa del Mar itself has relatively few places for young people to meet and interact, and certainly far fewer bars, parks, and billiard halls than Villa del Sol. However, the town does have a long, attractive beach; it is used as a meeting place during the day and a place for discreet lovemaking at night.

Although this discussion might lead one to conclude that there is not really that much to differentiate the sexual geographies of the two communities, those differences that do exist are significant, and hold important implications for the sexual lives of the young people involved. Particularly salient in this regard is the fact that while Villa del Sol has many well-defined leisure spaces (e.g., coffee houses, the city square, and so forth), in Villa del Mar young people's principal hangout is the street itself, which leaves adults with little scope to monitor or control the activities of their children.

Needless to say, certain dangers are inherent in young people's use of the street in this way. Not only is there little oversight by police or other authority figures, but the threat of violence (including sexual violence) is omnipresent. The fact that the street is shared with a large population of pushers and addicts ensures that drugs, including crack cocaine, are always available to those who are tempted to try them. Also relevant in this regard is the large number of foreign tourists who come to the town, attracted by its tropical mystique and "exotic" young bodies. Thus, there is always scope for young people of both sexes to earn some extra money by providing sexual services to foreigners staying in town. As one might imagine, there are no such possibilities in Villa del Sol, where community vigilance and a suspicion of strangers serve to dissuade outsiders from attempting to proposition or sell drugs to the young people of the town.

We have already referred to the sexual anonymity that San José affords to the youth of Villa del Sol. Should they wish to find a gay lover, harass transvestites dressed in drag, or take part in a discreet affair, they need merely board a bus, safe in the assumption that their friends and family back home will never find out. Such anonymity is unheard-of in Villa del Mar, where young people can be sure that news of their every move, their every sexual peccadillo will eventually get back to those they know. Thus, there is little scope for girls to practice prostitution or gays and lesbians to meet prospective mates without it becoming common knowledge.

Of course, one of the consequences of this state of affairs is the fact that young people in Villa del Mar cannot help but be exposed to a wide range of human sexual activity. That is to say, not only do many of them enjoy personal acquaintance with child molesters, transvestites, gay men, lesbians, *cacheros,** pimps, and sex trade workers, but they are likely to be more tolerant of sexual difference as a result. This stands in marked contrast to Villa del Sol, where one's sexual predilections are kept well hidden, and young people are unlikely ever to meet an openly gay individual. Needless to say, the apparent absence of sexual "deviance" from the community serves to create an environment ripe for the condemnation and criticism of sexual "others."

In Villa del Mar the home itself becomes a site for youthful sexual practice, a product of the frequency with which children are left alone by working mothers and absentee fathers. Not only does this provide young people with the opportunity to engage in illicit affairs, but it also facilitates sexual abuse by family members. This is less common in Villa del Sol, where the nuclear family remains

---

Cachero is a term used to describe men who have sex with other men, yet self-identify as heterosexual.

the norm, and stay-at-home mothers limit opportunities for sexual activity of any sort.

Similar differences are observable in the communities' respective high schools. In Villa del Mar, for example, where relatively little stock is placed in formal education, young people tend to see secondary school primarily as a prelude to work or marriage (certainly not university), with adolescent girls in particular hoping that it will provide a venue for meeting their husband-to-be, and hence an opportunity to leave their parents' home. As one might imagine, this orientation renders female high school students in Villa del Mar far more likely to engage in sex with their male counterparts than is the case in Villa del Sol. Here, most young women (and young men) expect to continue their education beyond the secondary level, and hence are extremely leery of any sexual relationship that may result in an unplanned pregnancy. In this way, both women and men tend to be quite careful in exercising their sexual choices, and generally do not establish strong emotional bonds during the course of their high school years.

Chapter 3

Methodology

ORGANIZATION OF THE STUDY

Initiated by the ILPES Research Department in January 1994, the present study was undertaken over a two-year period, with the final report being completed in December 1995. Figure 3.1 summarizes the structure of the research team.

Overall control of project execution was initially placed in the hands of two research directors. However, given the complexities

FIGURE 3.1. Organization of the Research Team

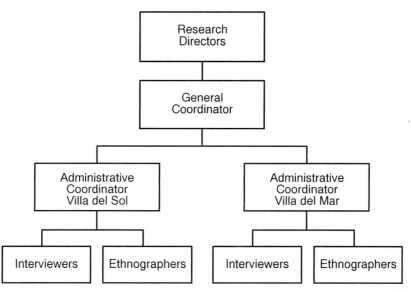

involved, it was deemed necessary to appoint a general coordinator who would take charge of all aspects of study implementation, including inventory management and preliminary review of the raw data (i.e., from interviews and focus groups). This individual was also responsible for the supervision of two administrative coordinators, one for each community, whose principal duties encompassed public relations, organization of focus groups, and identification of key informants and people who would carry out the in-depth interviews. Meanwhile, ethnographers participated in the day-to-day activities of young people, as well as conducting focus groups and interviews with community leaders.

SPECIFIC OBJECTIVES

As stated previously, our principal aim in carrying out this study was to explore sexual culture as learned and internalized by Costa Rican youth, and to assess its impact upon sexual practice and the risk of HIV infection. In turn, this provided the basis for the development of seven concrete research objectives:

1. To identify predominant sexual discourses, whether formal or informal in orientation
2. To assess the credibility and coherence of these discourses
3. To explore discourses' contradictions and inconsistencies, as well as the pressures they exert on individuals
4. Based on the above, to assess the relationship between sexual culture and young people's sexual practice, specifically with reference to the risk posed by HIV infection
5. To develop a conceptual model of the sexual cultures of Costa Rican youth that could serve as the basis for future interventions in the field of prevention
6. To assess the impact of newly emergent (nontraditional) sexual discourses, such as those associated with the spread of Protestant fundamentalism
7. To explore the role of misogyny and sex-based stereotyping in the context of young people's sexuality

TARGET POPULATION AND STUDY SAMPLE

Having decided that our target population would consist of young people of both sexes who were longtime residents of either Villa del Mar or Villa del Sol, we set about the task of elaborating a sample of young people (ages twelve to nineteen) drawn from both communities. This age bracket was chosen because it encompasses the period when profound changes take place in the lives of young people, including (inter alia) first sexual experience and first menstruation.

A series of quotas were used to generate the sample, with community membership, sex, age, first sexual experience, and onset of menstruation (for girls) being the principal criteria. In total, fifty-six individuals were selected, and were characterized by the set of attributes shown in Tables 3.1 and 3.2.

TABLE 3.1. Study Sample Broken Down by Age and Sex

	Villa del Mar			Villa del Sol		
Age	Males	Females	Total	Males	Females	Total
12-14	7	7	14	3	3	6
15-17	5	6	11	7	13	20
18-19	1	2	3	2	0	2
Total	13	15	28	12	16	28

TABLE 3.2. Study Sample Broken Down by Sex and Age of First Sexual Experience

Age	Villa del Mar					Villa del Sol				
	When did you have your first sexual experience?									
	Males		Females		Total	Males		Females		Total
Age	Yes	No	Yes	No		Yes	No	Yes	No	
12-14	0	7	1	6	14	0	3	0	3	6
15-17	4	1	3	3	11	2	5	3	10	20
18-19	0	1	0	2	3	0	2	0	0	2
Total	4	9	4	11	28	2	10	3	13	28

As Table 3.2 suggests, the majority of young people—of both sexes—had had no sexual experience prior to their inclusion in the sample. However, the nature of the study was such that this did not prevent us from gathering sufficient information about those who were sexually experienced.

Table 3.3 outlines the age at which girls in the sample had their first menstruation:

TABLE 3.3. Study Sample Broken Down by Age of First Menstruation

	Villa del Mar			Villa del Sol		
	When did you have your first menstruation?					
Age	Yes	No	Total	Yes	No	Total
12-14	5	3	8	2	2	4
15-17	5	0	5	12	0	12
18-19	2	0	2	0	0	0
Total	12	3	15	14	2	16

RESEARCH METHODS

Given the importance of the in-depth, qualitative interviews to the ultimate success of the project, considerable investment was made to ensure that they were carried out in an appropriate fashion. Consultants were hired to provide training to the interviewers and to assist in the preparation of an interview guide.

In addition to the interviews, participant observation was also incorporated into the methodology of this study. It provided a means of obtaining information about youth and their sexual practices in a nonthreatening, unobtrusive manner. To carry out these observations, project ethnographers frequented the bars, discotheques, beaches, and others places where young people gather. They also participated in religious, cultural, and sporting events, and recorded key details concerning the nature and location of youngsters' activities.

A series of focus groups were also carried out by field staff. These provided a means of obtaining additional information about young people's sexual culture, while at the same time serving to corroborate the findings of project ethnographers and interviewers. In this way, they were helpful in casting further light upon each community's social milieu, as well as the nature of young people's relationships, lifestyles, and emotions.

PREPARATION OF AN INTERVIEW GUIDE

Based on a guide we drew up to assist those who were charged with carrying out the in-depth interviews, the interviewers were subjected to three series of tests: first during initial training of staff; second during the project pilot; and third during the final training workshop (see Table 3.4).

TABLE 3.4. Timetable of Activities

Activities	1994												1995											
	1	2	3	4	5	6	7	8	9	10	11	12	1	2	3	4	5	6	7	8	9	10	11	12
Phase 1: Scoping; Preparation	▓	▓																						
Training of interviewers		▓																						
Visits to communities			▓																					
Recruitment of interview participants				▓																				
Pilot study					▓																			
Report on pilot study						▓																		
Modification of interview guide						▓																		
Modification of project methodology						▓																		
Final training workshop for interviewers							▓																	
Phase 2: Data collection; In-depth interviews							▓	▓	▓	▓	▓	▓	▓	▓	▓	▓								
Focus groups								▓	▓	▓	▓	▓	▓	▓	▓	▓	▓	▓						
Interviews with key informants								▓	▓	▓	▓	▓	▓	▓	▓	▓	▓	▓						
Participant observation									▓	▓	▓	▓	▓	▓	▓	▓	▓	▓						

TABLE 3.4 *(continued)*

Activities	1994 1	2	3	4	5	6	7	8	9	10	11	12	1995 1	2	3	4	5	6	7	8	9	10	11	12
Transcription of interviews											▓	▓	▓	▓	▓	▓	▓							
Interim report																		▓						
Phase 3: Data analysis														▓	▓	▓	▓							
Preparation of final report																					▓	▓		
Translation into English																							▓	▓

In essence, the interview guide provided a list of questions on a wide range of topics (e.g., religion, gender relations, family, sex, education, bodily perceptions, and so forth), whose underlying purpose was to elicit information about sexual discourses, their inter-relationships and contradictions, along with young people's resistance to them. The specific issues addressed by the guide are summarized as follows.

Questions Related to Formal Sexual Discourses and Their Impact on Young People (in the Home, on the Street, at School)

1. What is the substance of sexual information and discourses to which young people are exposed in the street, in the home, and at school? What principles, norms, ideals, behaviors, and practices do they promote? How do they vary among the two communities?
2. What differences distinguish one discourse from another, and what are their contradictions? To the extent that discourses promote different practices depending upon individuals' gender or religion, how might one characterize their variable impact upon those who benefit and those suffer from them most?
3. How might one characterize young people's perception of discourses, along with their norms, rules, principles, and objectives? How do young people respond to the latter? How are messages internalized and how do they influence young people's sexual life?

4. What is the role of such external factors as unemployment, drug addiction, sexual abuse, divorce, and abandonment, and how do they influence young people's sexuality and their view of the world?

Questions Related to Christian Fundamentalist Discourse and Its Impact on Sexuality

1. How does this discourse influence young people's sexuality?
2. What is the relationship between this discourse and nonfundamentalist sexual discourses, and what implications (if any) do their interactions hold for young people?

Questions Related to Sexism in Costa Rica and Its Influence on Sex Education in Schools

1. How, when, and for what reason are sexist discourses established in Costa Rican society?
2. What are the consequences of sexism? These may include, but are not limited to, sex-based discrimination, sexual aggression, sexual precocity, prostitution, and unsafe sexual practices.
3. What factors are significant in reinforcing or undermining sexism and double standards among different groups of young people?
4. How does sexism influence young people's view and practice of sex, and to what extent are variables such as age, gender, class, religion, place of residence, and education significant in this regard?
5. What is the relationship between sexual stereotyping, knowledge of AIDS, and the practice of safe sex among men and women?
6. What could be done to counter sexism and sexual violence among young people, and promote a healthier, more equitable relationship between men and women?

Questions Related to the Interrelationship Between Discourses and Activities That Place Individuals at High Risk of Contracting HIV

1. In what ways does practice differ from theory and how do young people sort out the contradictions and inconsistencies that may be inherent within dominant discourses?

2. To what extent does sexual expression and understanding vary along lines of age, gender, place of residence, religion, and social class?
3. What factors are at work in inducing young people to engage in, or refrain from engaging in, sexual intercourse? Relevant factors may include, but are not limited to, parties, religion, substance use, peer pressure, sexual aggression, economic problems, parental influence, sex education, and myths.
4. In what contexts is the pressure to engage in sexual intercourse most strongly felt?

Needless to say, the quantity of data gathered during the course of the interview process was enormous. However, rather than attempting to condense the material through interviewer syntheses or the preparation of case histories, we deemed it crucial that the young people be allowed to speak for themselves. Otherwise, we were afraid that the conservative nature of Costa Rican society, particularly in relation to adolescent sexuality, would cause people to disbelieve or reject our findings.

SELECTION AND TRAINING OF INTERVIEWERS

Given the key role played by the interviewer in the qualitative research process, considerable time and resources were devoted to the task of recruiting appropriate field staff. In the paragraphs below we summarize some of the issues taken into account as we embarked upon this exercise.

First, it was essential that interviewers be able to display an appropriate degree of sensitivity to research participants. While acknowledging that a postsecondary education is no guarantee of this sensitivity, we felt that by focusing our recruitment campaign on university campuses, our field staff would at the very least be likely to possess the background necessary to conduct the interviews in a professional manner. Any gaps in interviewers' knowledge base would be corrected through specialized training.

Second, it was considered likely that the interview process would arouse strong emotions on the part of some participants, particularly if they had suffered sexual, physical, or psychological abuse in the past. Thus, as part of their training, field staff (many of whom were upper-level psychology students) were taught crisis intervention techniques and given a list of professionals to whom participants could be referred.

Finally, it was emphasized to us by our consultants during training exercises that young people would be extremely leery of discussing personal matters with fellow community members, and that they would prefer to be interviewed by people they did not know.

As one might imagine, these considerations forced us to look beyond the communities themselves for suitable interview staff. Had we not planned for this contingency from the outset, the costs involved could have been prohibitive, but as it was the administrative coordinator was able to facilitate the process through judicious management of interview logistics.

During the first phase of project implementation (February 1994), approximately ten individuals were trained to conduct interviews and engage in other research-related activities. This group was subsequently given the task of carrying out a pilot study. It was on the basis of this pilot that we reviewed the overall feasibility of the study itself (May and June 1994), and subsequently made the decision to train a larger group of interviewers, so as to save time and extend the project's scope (July 1994).

To expedite the recruitment of additional staff, a circular was prepared and distributed to all Costa Rican universities. Résumés were received from roughly thirty undergraduate and graduate students, from which we selected twenty individuals between the ages of twenty-two and twenty-six. Hiring criteria included a strong academic record, proven ability to handle responsibility, interest in the study, and willingness to travel. To ensure that study participants did not feel alienated by their interviewer, class background and gender were also taken into account by the hiring committee.

Upon selection, field staff were asked to participate in a one-week training course. A range of issues were addressed during the course, including presentation of the basic tenets of postmodernism (social constructionism, discourse theory, and relevant methodologies), religious fundamentalism (sociohistorical context, analysis of fundamentalist sexual discourses, and forms of resistance by young people), and the gender-sex dichotomy (feminist theory and conceptualizations of masculinity).

The internalization of sexual discourses by project participants was also addressed in the training workshop, as were the forms of resistance these discourses may engender and their likely impact upon the interview process. Field staff also engaged in practice interviews, feedback from which resulted in further modifications to the interview guide.

PROCESS OF CONDUCTING IN-DEPTH INTERVIEWS

The first step in project implementation involved publicizing the study in the two communities, followed by a series of reconnaissance visits to carry out ethnographic observation and interviews with community leaders. With the help of the administrative coordinator in each town, key sites and institutions were visited in order to compile relevant data on young people's leisure activities, along with their behavior, emotions, and ways of thinking. Initial probing in the area of sexual discourses also took place at this time.

The first in-depth interviews were conducted in Villa del Mar in July 1994. The administrative coordinator in this community, well-respected for her work in the health sector, made initial contact with young people, as well as explaining the nature of the project to their parents. All interviews were tape-recorded and, as a way of building trust between field staff and participants, men were only interviewed by men, and women by women. Sessions lasted anywhere from six to eight hours, generally broken up into three or four two-hour segments.

Approximately one month later (in August 1994), interviews began in Villa del Sol, with officials of a local secondary school permitting use of the facilities for this purpose. As was the case in Villa del Mar, interview logistics were handled by the town's administrative coordinator, a psychologist who was also a resident of the community.

Between July 1994 and March 1995, fifty-six interviews were successfully carried out in the two towns (twenty-eight in each). Significantly, only three individuals (two men and a woman)—all from Villa del Sol—decided to bow out in the midst of the interview process. Clearly, the high level of dedication and enthusiasm of field staff played a key role in ensuring the interviews' success.

FOCUS GROUPS

On the basis of initial findings from the interviews, it was decided to hold a series of group sessions to cast additional light upon a number of ambiguous or otherwise underexplored issues. For the most part, these topics had previously been identified in the interview guide and were related to the sexual lives of young people, conceptualizations of femininity and masculinity, entertainment and leisure activities, community problems, HIV/AIDS, and relationships with parents, peers, and significant others. Two focus groups of roughly three hours in length were also held with young members of fundamentalist churches in both communities.

All of these sessions were taped. In Villa del Mar, focus groups were held over the course of four weekends in November and December 1994, with men and women meeting separately in groups of ten. Once again, the administrative coordinator was responsible for making all necessary arrangements, including rental of the town's community hall. Particularly noteworthy in this regard is the fact that one of the groups was made up primarily of members of a Roman Catholic youth organization, none of whom had participated in an in-depth interview.

Focus groups were also carried out in Villa del Sol, albeit with greater difficulty due to the reluctance of some youths to participate in this type of activity. Thanks to the efforts of the local project coordinator, groups sessions were eventually held, and were organized along lines similar to those of Villa del Mar. Meeting places included the community's Red Cross office and a private home.

However, it should be noted that, due to the reluctance of Villa del Sol youth to take part in the focus group sessions, we were forced to approach a number of local religious organizations to help us carry them out. This in turn meant that most group members were drawn from the ranks of these organizations, which prompted us to drop the subject of religion, given that the views expressed would likely not be representative of the entire community in any case. Instead, we relied on findings derived from the in-depth, personal interviews.

Focus groups were facilitated by men and women who had previously worked on the project as interviewers or ethnographers. These individuals made use of a range of techniques to elicit participants' views and responses, with particular emphasis placed upon participatory approaches. Examples of the latter include role-play (to explore men and women's understanding of themselves and each other) and visualization exercises (to identify and make sense of sex-based stereotypes). Facilitators also asked participants to break into smaller groups to discuss issues such as homosexuality, virginity, and gender relations.

We were also interested in determining whether young people's behavior differed when confronted with mixed- or single-sex groups. When the sessions were mixed, we generally found that women were less willing to voice their opinions, particularly on the subject of sex. Meanwhile, young men were most anxious when they were among other males, leading us to conclude that they needed women present to protect them from intimate questioning of a sort that would force them to reveal their innermost feelings in front of male peers.

INTERVIEWS WITH COMMUNITY LEADERS

It has already been noted that Villa del Mar community leaders were far more receptive to our requests for interviews than were those in Villa del Sol (see Table 3.5), where a local priest spoke out against our work in the area. Among those whom we interviewed were school teachers, church officials (including priests and ministers), bar owners, health care workers, drug dealers, politicians, civil servants, nongovernmental organization staffers, and business people.

TABLE 3.5. Interviews with Community Leaders Broken Down by Community

Community	Men	Women	Total
Villa del Mar	9	6	15
Villa del Sol	1	2	3
Total	10	8	18

TRANSCRIPTION AND DATA ANALYSIS

Transcription proved to be an arduous task due to the length and number of interviews carried out. Taking roughly five months to complete, from December 1994 to April 1995, the material was entered into a custom-designed data management program called SAPAC. In essence, the program allows users to codify and sort information while it is on the screen in front of them.

A team of three researchers engaged in an initial round of data analysis to identify the most salient issues and themes. This was followed by a second round of more intensive exploration, involving the shuffling and reshuffling of material as a means of teasing out key patterns and contradictions. Needless to say, the sheer volume of interview and focus group material prevented us from analyzing it in highly detailed terms. Nevertheless, our conceptual framework, discussed at length in Chapter 4, provided a powerful lens through which to make sense of the data.

METHODOLOGICAL CHALLENGES

Given the nature of this study, it is not particularly surprising that members of the interview team were themselves faced with certain difficulties in coming to terms with the subject matter. Not only were few familiar with the concept of social constructionism, but most had never engaged in a truly frank discussion of such contentious issues as male violence and sexism.

Thus, during the course of the training workshops it was decided that, if young people were to speak openly about their sexuality, field staff should be expected to do the same. This in turn provided the basis for a series of candid and often painful admissions by team members as they delved into their memories and innermost emotions. Significantly, not only did this self-reflectivity contribute to interviewers' ability to handle difficult or controversial topics in the interviews themselves, but several indicated to us that the training workshops had also helped them sort out problems they were dealing with in their own lives.

It should be noted as well that a number of changes were made to the project methodology once the implementation process had begun. In the first instance, research directors were forced to change the order of interventions, so that the in-depth interviews were held before the group sessions rather than the reverse (as had originally been foreseen). This decision was made for several reasons, including, most notably, problems in recruiting a sufficient number of workshop facilitators, along with young people's initial reluctance to discuss personal issues in a group setting.

Difficulties were also encountered during the ethnographic phase of the study. While it had been our hope prior to the initiation of field work that the ethnographers would take part in a wide range of community activities, in fact much of their time was spent conducting personal interviews. As one might imagine, this left us with a significant gap in our knowledge of key issues in young people's lives, which we sought to address through a series of meetings with focus group facilitators and the two community coordinators.

Meanwhile, on a purely logistical level, field workers were faced with a series of challenges in scheduling group sessions in the two communities. Although they had originally planned to recruit focus group participants from among those who had taken part in a personal interview, it was subsequently discovered that this would not always be feasible, due to young people's conflicting work, school, and social commitments. Thus, as a way of resolving this problem, sessions were held with members of already-established groups, such as church-based youth organizations.

As for the personal interviews themselves, there can be little doubt that the delicate nature of the subject matter addressed did not facilitate the recruitment of participants. Young people's reluctance to become involved was especially marked in Villa del Sol, where three individuals refused outright to participate, while others became wary after hearing some of the questions to be asked from members of earlier sessions.

Finally, it must be acknowledged that we never successfully resolved the problem posed by Villa del Sol community leaders' refusal to support the project. Field staff were only able to secure interviews with three such individuals; others excused themselves by saying they had no time, or, in less diplomatic fashion, that they simply did not want to cooperate. It is thought that the community's priest, who initially supported our work but later decided to oppose it, may have been influential in these decisions. Still, this is not to suggest that our field workers faced no obstacles in Villa del Mar. In particular, interviewers, facilitators, and ethnographers often had to contend with personal safety concerns, given the high risk of being robbed or assaulted in some of the neighborhoods in which they worked. That they managed to avoid being victimized in this way was in large measure due to the guidance and advice provided by our community coordinator, who was familiar with local conditions and well-respected by community members because of her work as a nurse.

Chapter 4

Conceptual Frame for the Analysis of Sexual Culture

INTRODUCTION TO SOCIAL CONSTRUCTIONISM

Social constructionism emerged in the 1970s as part of a wider reaction against dominant Western sexual "norms," and it encompasses a range of theoretical (and political) perspectives. Discussed at length by Carole Vance (1991) in her article, "Anthropology Rediscovers Sexuality: A Theoretical Comment," it is clear that feminists have been among the movement's most forceful proponents. For example, Gayle Rubin has written several papers that explore the notion of a "sex-gender system," in which biological characteristics and social relations are collapsed into a single explanatory framework, regardless of the fact that they are both driven by quite different dynamics. Once this is understood, women's subordination ceases to be a mere accident of biology, and becomes grounded instead in the social structures—and systems of domination—that surround us (Vance, 1991).

Also significant in this regard is the work on sexuality carried out by scholars such as Weeks and Foucault. To summarize what is admittedly a highly complex set of arguments, these writers argue that homosexuality emerged in the nineteenth century in response to a particular set of sociohistorical conditions. That is to say, it was only through the development of modern psychiatry that an attempt was made to ground certain physical acts in an overarching sexual identity (Weeks, 1977). Needless to say, the significance of these conclusions was not lost upon those who were working with the hidden biographies of gays and lesbians from the last century. For these individuals, questions regarding the origins of homosexuality had long perplexed them. Have the categories "gay" and "lesbian" always existed? If not, when and how did they develop? What processes underlie the imbuing of identical physical acts with highly divergent sexual meanings (Vance, 1991)?

Through their engagement with these questions, writers became increasingly cognizant of the cultural underpinnings of supposedly immutable sexual categories (i.e., heterosexual, bisexual, or homosexual). Moreover, nowhere was this more obvious than in the work that explored the relationship between sexual practice and sexual culture in different historical periods (Weeks, 1979). Ancient Greeks, for example, made no distinction between heterosexuality and homosexuality, only between activity and passivity. In this way, men were deemed "active" to the extent that they penetrated others, regardless of whether these others were men, women, slaves, or free. As one might imagine, these findings serve to confirm the view that, rather than being born with a particular set of sexual characteristics, human beings acquire their sexual identity through socialization, with sexual culture playing a crucial role in informing and underpinning this learning process.

However, it should be emphasized that the importance of social constructionism lies not merely in its ability to shed light upon the historical dimensions of sexuality, but also in its relevance to present-day analyses of sex, power, and the state. In short, the modern era has been characterized by the progressive encroachment of state and parastate agencies (e.g., physicians, social workers, scientists) on the personal lives of citizens, usurping the Church's power to determine who is normal and who is "deviant" in the process. In this way, constructionism provides a basis upon which to explore the articulation of sexual discourses with the political agendas of a range of social actors, including church and state.

BASIC PRINCIPLES

While acknowledging that social constructionism is a broad church, encompassing a wide array of writers and positions, it is nonetheless possible to identify several areas of convergence.

In the first instance, constructionists agree that sexuality is grounded in social factors and not, as essentialists pretend, in the natural world (Vance, 1991). Needless to say, this implies a rejection of the notion that instinct determines certain types of behavior, such as women's "need" to nurture. This conclusion was reached in the wake of transcultural behavioral studies that highlighted the remarkable degree of geographic variance in people's understanding of masculinity and femininity. In short, not only did these studies find evidence of cultural contexts in which nurturing was *not* associated with women, but they also documented many cases in which men were engaged in behavior that, while "normal" in their own eyes, would be considered highly effeminate in Europe or the Americas (Laumann and Laumann, 1994). Driven by findings such as these, constructionist scholars were led to argue that individuals' sexual behavior can only be explained with reference to the particular social system in which they find themselves.

Closely related to this last point is the constructionist view that any number of subjective meanings may be attributed to a single physical act, depending upon the particular cultural context in which it manifests itself (Vance, 1991). Thus, as Gagnon (1977) makes clear, one should be extremely wary of imposing one's own understanding of sexual behavior upon other times and other cultures. For example, ancient pagan religious rites involving gay sexual practice were not considered "abnormal" at the time. Along similar lines, even though sodomy was strongly condemned in medieval Europe, this did not mean that individuals were categorized according to their sexual orientation. In short, before the nineteenth century, any man could engage in sodomy with a woman, man, or animal without being labeled "homosexual" (Weeks, 1985). Given the extent to which this view differs from that which is predominant in the West today, constructionists would argue that each culture develops its own means of naming and classifying the sexual and emotional experiences of its members.

Indeed, many believe that individuals' determination of sexual pleasure is itself influenced by cultural factors. For example, despite the fact that gynecological or breast examinations may involve behavior that is reminiscent of the sex act, they do not produce pleasure because of the context in which they are carried out. Similarly, most prepubescent girls do not consider their breasts to be erogenous zones. Having realized that boys find them attractive, they begin to see them in a different light as well. In contrast, the fact that boys' nipples and breasts are often highly sensitive to the touch is quickly suppressed in cultures where this type of arousal is deemed "unmasculine."

Adopting an even more radical stance, some constructionists argue that sexual desire itself is socially determined (Vance, 1991), citing the degree of variance in what is considered attractive (and hence sexually arousing) over time and space. Indeed, a number of writers have even sought to include sexual orientation in this regard, asserting that individuals' homosexual or heterosexual identity is less the product of genetic predisposition, and more of socialization. Thus, whereas Western sexual culture has traditionally left little scope for the adoption of alternative sexual identities, other cultures may be far less prescriptive.

SEXUAL DISCOURSES

Having endeavored to lay bare the social bases of human sexuality, we now turn to the means by which sexual culture is internalized, that is, through sexual discourses. These refer to all the ideas, principles, and myths related to sexuality that characterize a particular society at a given moment in its history, with an individual's sexual behavior determined by the manner in which he or she assimilates them.

As discussed in previous chapters, sexual discourses can either be formal or informal in orientation. While the former tend to be promoted by (and serve the interests of) official institutions, including most notably the state, the latter offer alternatives or challenges to dominant ways of thinking, and are generally associated with less powerful strata of society, including oppositional social movements. As one might imagine, formal discourses include those informed by scientific rationality (whether in the guise of medicine, psychiatry, or sexology), religion, or the state (through legislation or the public education system), while informal discourses may be rooted in feminism (whether radical or liberal) or in the tenets of romantic love.

Not surprisingly, sexual discourses are also present at the interpersonal level, encompassing both face-to-face communication between individuals (whether parent and child, physician and patient, teacher and student, or priest and parishioner), and messages mediated through television, music, and the visual arts.

Still, this is not to suggest that sexual discourses enjoy an autonomous existence. Indeed, nothing could be further from the truth, given the extent to which they are constituted and reproduced by the daily "discursive practices" of individuals themselves. How so? Quite simply, it is these practices—which include anything from the color of young girls' clothing to male sexual violence—that are responsible for actualizing a particular discourse, and for ensuring that it continues to exist through time. It is also through such practices that discourses are modified, which occurs when a given practice is confronted with a sufficient degree of contradiction or resistance in the "real" world of social relations and social life.

It is possible to characterize sexual discourses, with reference to the following points:

1. They are socially normative. Discourses aim to define sexuality and govern the contexts in which it is expressed, as well the partners with whom one may legitimately pursue sexual relations. Such discourses also purport to circumscribe their relationship with other spheres of social activity, providing explanations of their overarching purpose and relevance in the process. For religious discourses, for example, sexuality is understood to be part of a divine plan, whereas those rooted in gender expound upon the importance of biology and natural selection.

2. They are coercive. Discourses forbid, discourage, and censure all that falls outside of their purpose, principles, and norms. Transgressors are punished through a variety of means, ranging from death and lifelong exile to ostracism and silent disapproval. While there may very well be wide variance in the control and surveillance mechanisms available to particular discourses, all exact a price for offenses committed against them, even if the punishment is merely self-inflicted.

3. They alternate between complementarity and contradiction. As has been emphasized previously, discourses are grounded in ideologies and worldviews in which sex is seen as merely one element of a larger whole. Gender discourses, for example, posit a system of

patriarchal domination in which women are exploited in a range of areas that include, but are not limited to, the field of sexuality. Along similar lines, Christian discourses encompass an understanding of life and death in which sex plays an integral role. Given that discourses also overlap, they are likely to address many of the same issues, including sex, in either a complementary or contradictory fashion. Thus, at the same time that Christian discourses call upon women to devote themselves to husband and home, romantic discourses do the same (albeit for different reasons), thereby generating a measure of complementarity. However, this in turn is undermined by the latter's acceptance of the view that allowances can be made for the sake of amorous passion, something that runs directly counter to the Christian emphasis upon self-sacrifice and chastity.

4. They are not seamless. That is to say, discourses are often characterized by a degree of internal contradiction or discongruity, whereby disconnected elements may very well promote conflicting behavior, attitudes, and values. To offer but one example, rational-scientific sexual discourses emerge from a range of disciplinary contexts, including demography, sexology, and medicine, among others. Each provides its own particular perspective (and prejudices): demography emphasizes age of first sexual relationship, contraceptive use, and population growth; sexology highlights the importance of sexual communication, sexual pleasure, and orgasm; while medicine focuses upon breast-feeding, STDs, and infant mortality.

5. They are exhaustive. Although this may seem to contradict previous statements, one must bear in mind that the messages inherent within a given discourse are communicated implicitly as well as explicitly. Thus, what is not said is just as important as what is. For example, individuals are left to infer the bounds of legitimate Christian sexuality by taking stock of what is *not* forbidden. Similarly, in gender discourses, men are defined with reference to what they are not, namely women.

6. They are dynamic, undergoing significant change in time and space. Thus, the same discourse may evolve in divergent ways in two locales, with perhaps the most obvious example being the way in which gender discourses differ widely in cities as compared to rural areas. Time is also significant in this regard, as is attested by the deep-seated changes wrought upon Christian sexuality in the past

2,000 years, as the early emphasis upon abstinence and self-denial were slowly replaced in subsequent centuries by a less hostile attitude toward sex.

7. They are never politically neutral. Inherent within any discourse is a system of power and knowledge whereby the interests of certain groups are promoted over those of others. In this way, one might argue that every discursive practice embodies a relationship of power, characterized either by the exercise of domination or resistance on the part of the actors involved.

8. They engender resistance. As Foucault (1978, Vol. 1) makes clear, power and resistance go hand in hand, with the application of the former necessarily calling forth the latter. Thus, even though all discourses embody a totalizing logic, this logic is always undermined by the counterstrategies and countertactics of those who benefit least from them.

SEXUAL PRACTICE AND IDENTITY

As is implicit in the previous discussion, discourses play a key role in the construction of sexual identities, that is, in the way that individuals define themselves vis à vis their physical bodies, objects of desire, and sexual practices.

At the most basic level, this is seen in the emphasis placed upon defining people according to their sexual partners. However, division of the world's population into discrete categories of heterosexuals, homosexuals, and bisexuals is of relatively recent vintage, closely associated with the spread of "Enlightenment" values in the eighteenth century, and the emergence of modern psychiatry in the nineteenth (Mahon, 1992; Weeks, 1985). Significantly, before this time class was seen as a far more important determinant of sexual identity. For the Greeks and Romans, for example, all individuals could be placed into one of two categories: active and free, or passive and enslaved. Thus, a free man could have sex with women or men, whether free or slaves and still remain a man, so long as he was the one who penetrated the other (Foucault, 1988, Vol. 3).

Modern sexual discourse has clearly had an effect in Costa Rica, where self-identification based on sexual orientation is now common among young people, particularly those living in urban areas. However, this is not to say that it has always been so. Before the 1960s, when the national government began to invest heavily in the industrial sector, most young people did not think of themselves in these terms. Rather, they drew upon the older categories of "active" and "passive," with men normally falling into the former while women were associated with the latter. Men who had sexual relations with other men and were "passive" in bed were thought of as women. Along similar lines, lesbians were categorized according to their relative "activity" (hence, they were men) or "passivity" (women) in the relationship. Also relevant in this regard was the growing importance placed upon feelings and fantasies. That is, dreams had little or no place in the premodern sexual universe. Individuals' identity was grounded in practice; thoughts and feelings were immaterial. However, with the introduction of psychoanalysis to Costa Rica in the 1950s, the ground began to shift, and the mind became an increasingly important site in the determination of "normal" sexual development and identity.

Still, even as one acknowledges the key role played by hegemonic discourses in shaping each individual's sexual identity, they are by no means the only forces at work. Other relevant factors include discourses' internal contradictions, economic and social marginalization, and scientific and technological innovation, as well as the resistance that dominant discourses always engender.

GENDER, IDENTITY, AND SEXUAL ROLES

Of all the sexual discourses, none is more important to the development of an individual's sexual identity than those centered on gender. From the moment babies are born, they are defined and categorized according to their sex. Indeed, as Kaschak (1993) argues, perceptions of babies' size, intelligence, and level of activity have all been shown to vary widely depending upon the sex to which they are thought to belong.

Given that gender discourses are not closely associated with a particular institution, be it the Roman Catholic Church or the scientific establishment, one may very well be surprised by their seeming durability. Yet one need only consider the degree to which they have been appropriated by other discourses, Christianity most notable among them, to appreciate their continuing importance and power.

Thus, despite the fact that traditional gender discourses may upon occasion undermine the existing social order, for the most part they sustain it, with two of the most significant means in this regard being sexual orientation and sexual role enforcement. As one might imagine, the former seeks to ensure that women and men "complement" one another by positing heterosexuality as the only legitimate expression of sexuality, while the latter provides individuals with norms for how they should act, feel, and express themselves. Needless to say, men as a group derive significant benefit from this gender system; they also help to sustain it, through their monopolization of the country's political, social, and economic resources.

It is important to note that gender discourses do not always manifest themselves in identical ways. For example, community members in Villa del Mar and Villa del Sol differ significantly in their understanding of "appropriate" sexual roles and orientation. In the former case, men and women are perceived as opposites, each with their own sphere of influence: the man provides for the family, while the woman takes care of the home. In the middle-class community, in contrast, women and men are understood to complement each other, meaning that women can engage in "masculine" activities (e.g., work outside the home), yet still be considered feminine.

Despite the crucial role played by gender discourses in shaping individuals' behavior and identity, one must be careful not to attribute to them the powers of a puppeteer, exercising total control over young people's minds and bodies. Rather, the bases of the existing gender order are negotiated on a daily basis by Costa Rican youth, who reshape it through their own interventions just as it reshapes them.

Still, this is not to say that its demise is in any way imminent. Indeed, nothing could be further from the truth. As our research in Villa del Sol has shown, the existing gender system can undergo change without threatening the fundamental power imbalance between men and women. Thus, regardless of the fact that the women of this community are now able to go to university and pursue a career, they are still the ones who do most of the work in the home, as well as providing emotional support to their partners. Because of this, one is left wondering how much they have advanced relative to their sisters in Villa del Mar, whose work duties do not extend beyond the front door of their homes.

DISCOURSES AND PREVENTION

Given the power of discourses to shape individuals' sexual identity and behavior, it should come as no surprise that they also play a crucial role in the transmission of attitudes and values that serve to facilitate the spread of HIV/AIDS in the population at large. Consider, for example, the case of Latin America's gender order: at the same time that women are roundly condemned should they wish to experiment sexually with multiple partners, men are actively encouraged to do so, if only to provide proof of their virility and prowess in bed. In this way, the extent to which married women are at risk of contracting HIV is more dependent upon their husbands' sexual activities than their own.

Thus, AIDS-prevention initiatives that do not pay adequate heed to existing sexual discourses (and power imbalances) are doomed to failure, with an obvious example being the condom campaign advocated by Costa Rica's scientific community. From the beginning, its effectiveness as a means of combating the AIDS epidemic has been undermined by the Roman Catholic Church on the one hand, which challenged the morality of this approach while recommending fidelity as a more suitable response, and dominant gender discourses on the other, which provide women with little scope to ensure that their partners use a condom during sex.

Faced with these disjunctures among the various discourses, individuals respond in a number of ways, not all of which contribute positively to the cause of AIDS prevention. For example, some respond to the Church's condemnation of extramarital affairs by engaging in anonymous sex with prostitutes in public places. Given the need for haste and discretion, measures designed to minimize the likelihood of infection are set aside in the name of pleasure.

Along somewhat different lines, compartmentalization also provides a way of dealing with discursive contradictions. In essence a coping strategy, it offers individuals a means of engaging in mutually incompatible practices or thought processes without calling into question the assumptions upon which their worldview is based. In this way, a young man who has internalized the Church's teachings on sex and sexuality is able to set them aside when he is in the company of his male friends far from home, or in any situation that calls for displays of sexual bravado and aggression on his part. Of course, this only serves to highlight the need for prevention initiatives that are flexible, and whose messages are tailored to the range of situations and locales in which young people's sexuality manifests itself.

POWER AND KNOWLEDGE ARTICULATED IN DISCOURSES

As Foucault makes clear, power and discourse are closely intertwined, with the latter implicated in the production (and reproduction) of countless power relations across time and space. Indeed, it is precisely for this reason that discourses are so influential in our lives, given that they structure our every thought and interaction. However, it bears emphasis that the power they wield is exerted from below rather than from above, at the "microstructural" level of the home and the individual. It should be noted as well that this power tends to be "productive" rather than "repressive" in orientation. That is, discourses are sustained less through recourse to coercive force, and more through the effective management and channeling of individuals' productive capacities, with Christianity's artistic legacy being a case in point.

Still, in seeking to come to terms with the durability of hegemonic discourses, it is important to distinguish between force and discipline. Although it is seldom necessary to make use of the former, the latter is deployed on a more or less continuous basis, both with those who transgress the law and, more importantly, to induce individuals to police themselves. As Foucault (1977) makes clear, not only does disciplinary power of this sort energize the productive capacities of the people, but it also transforms them into "docile bodies," easily monitored and controlled.

Among the forces involved in this institutionalization process, none is more important than the state itself, enjoying as it does the capacity to intervene in almost all facets of social life, from the economy to the criminal justice system. However, this is not to say that all other actors are insignificant by comparison, with the Church and mass media being but two examples of institutions intimately involved in the task of shaping and structuring our understanding of sex and sexuality.

Underpinning the latter's work in this regard are microscale processes unfolding at the level of the family and individual. Not only do parents, children, and extended family members play a crucial role in policing one another's sexual behavior, but individuals, having internalized the discursive "rules of the game," are generally adept at disciplining themselves, controling their desires, and silencing "inappropriate" expressions of their sexuality (Foucault, 1983b, Vol. 2).

Recognizing the significance of these micropower relations within the larger context of hegemonic sexual discourse, this study endeavors—following Foucault's example—to analyze power from the bottom up. Thus, by paying attention to the means by which young people learn discourses, how they internalize them, and how they contribute to their reproduction, we hope to gain a deeper understanding of the particular relationship between the microscale and generalized systems of oppression (e.g., along lines of gender or class). Of course, in undertaking this project, it is critical that one avoid positing a binary opposition between oppressors and oppressed. Instead, power should be understood as decentered and ubiquitous, flowing through individuals, families, and institutions in constantly shifting terms.

HOW DO DISCOURSES ON SEX EMERGE?

With few exceptions, the hegemonic sexual discourses of the modern era are all rooted in eighteenth-century Europe, a period which Foucault (1978, Vol. 1) believes to be characterized by a significant shift in the relationship between state and citizen. In short, he argues that it was at this time that rulers ceased to see their people as a collection of individuals, and began to conceptualize them instead as a *population* possessing specific attributes and problems in need of intervention.

Sex was at the heart of this new understanding. If a country's population was to remain economically productive and politically docile, all matters pertaining to human reproduction had to be carefully monitored and controlled, including most notably the means by which individuals exercised their sexuality. In this way, sexual behavior became both an object of analysis and a site for intervention, with moral and religious exhortations, surveillance by state agents, and fiscal measures being only some of the tools deployed to promote family stability and a sustainable level of procreation.

It was also at this time that child and adolescent sexuality became an object of "serious" research. Not only were any number of treatises prepared on such topics as youthful masturbation and its consequences, but the medical establishment became increasingly interested in the study (and treatment) of "nervous illnesses," laying the groundwork for subsequent elaboration of the categories "sexual perversions" and "sexual crimes," beloved by psychiatrists and the criminal justice system respectively. Needless to say, with the deployment of each new category, new webs of power relations were created, along with the bureaucratic infrastructure necessary to monitor, investigate, treat, and confine all those who fell outside the bounds of the normal. Growing attention was also focused upon "prevention," that is, developing the tools needed to predict sexual abnormalities (e.g., through the accumulation of case histories and the like), while "educating" the public regarding the ubiquity of "sex criminals" in their neighborhoods and cities.

DISCOURSE INTERNALIZATION

As one might imagine, feedback is integral to the process of discourse internalization, which serves to foster a sexual culture which is itself implicated in the reproduction of hegemonic sexual discourses. Indeed, it is precisely in this way that sexualities come to reflect dominant societal values and thought processes.

At the most basic level, children "learn" sexuality under the guidance of their parents and families, who draw upon techniques ranging from repetition to inculcate them with an appropriate sexual outlook and value system. As for cases where these interventions fail to have their desired effect, more coercive methods are used, including manipulation, abandonment, physical assault, and—last but certainly not least—induced confession.

For Foucault, confession has long been one of the principal means by which dominant sexual values are communicated and enforced. Still, this is not to say that the institution has remained unchanged over the centuries. Originally deployed only in the context of penitence and absolution, since the eighteenth century it has become a key element within any number of structured relationships, with notable examples including teachers and pupils, doctors and patients, judges and defendants.

Thus, by way of summary, one might argue that successful discourse learning depends first upon the elaboration of a sexual culture that reflects the discourse in question, and second upon the structuring of individuals' consciences in a manner that renders them amenable to the internalization of the latter.

HOW ARE DISCOURSES IMPOSED?

Still, knowledge of the content of a given sexual discourse is in itself no guarantee that individuals will engage in behavior that is compatible with it. Rather, its precepts must be anchored in each person's mind through a number of structuring mechanisms. While acknowledging that many such mechanisms are at work within each individual, we touch upon five of the most important here:

1. *Repression* is used as a way of erasing or silencing deviant thoughts (e.g., feelings of pleasure when imagining violent sex) and memories (e.g., homosexual attractions).
2. Having been taught as children to feel *fear* in the face of "inappropriate" expressions of sexuality, individuals learn to associate particular acts and thoughts with the sense that they are in imminent physical danger.
3. *Shame* is another programmed response that is routinely invoked in individuals who think they have acted in an undignified manner or improperly exposed their bodies. This latter point is especially significant, underlining as it does the radical separation of the body into public and private domains, with the latter being associated with desire and all things dirty and base.

4. Along similar lines, *guilt* has also come to be closely associated with sexuality. Essentially a means of enforcing conformity, it induces us to act as our own judge, jury, and executioner, all the while forestalling inappropriate behavior by reminding us of the punishment that awaits us at the hands of our parents, our teachers, or God himself.

5. An individual feels *disgust* when he or she inadvertently swallows something repulsive, with the judgment, "This is not edible" becoming a frantic shout of "I must purge myself of it!" In matters of sexuality, this defense mechanism provides the basis for the rejection of certain acts and practices, particularly those of an oral or anal nature. Society's message is clear: "If you do not manage to steer clear of these impulses, you'll have to spit and vomit."

In this way, one might argue that discourse internalization is to a significant degree dependent upon processes of association, whereby certain social practices become articulated with basic physiological responses to unpleasant situations. Needless to say, not only does this serve to naturalize socially constructed categories and values, but it serves to reinforce—in highly evocative terms—societal aversion to "deviant" sexual practices.

CONTRADICTIONS INHERENT WITHIN SEXUAL DISCOURSES

As we have sought to argue, power presupposes resistance. That is, to the extent that power relations are imbued with the desire to dominate or compel obedience, they will inevitably call forth counterstrategies and countertactics on the part of dominated groups. Although the latter may take on any number of forms, one means of resistance involves the promotion of alternative discourses based upon premises that contradict those of their hegemonic counterparts.

From this perspective, contradiction serves to create a link between two discursive proposals whereby the verity of one demands the falsity of the other, as both cannot coexist at the same time. How so? On the one hand, there are cases in which individuals are called upon to adhere to opposing requirements, for example to refrain from sex prior to marriage (Christian discourse), and to become sexually active at an early age (street discourse).

On the other hand, there may also be a contradiction between discourses' requirements and individuals' capacity to fulfill them. This is often seen in poor neighborhoods where people have internalized the ideal of a permanent and lifelong marriage, yet their level of social and economic marginalization is such that they have no way of realizing this goal. In the event, psychological and material resources play a key role in shaping each person's response to discursive contradiction, with higher self-esteem and a more favorable socioeconomic status greatly facilitating the successful resolution of such conflicts.

Other examples of contradiction include those which arise from a disjuncture between theory and practice. Thus, while both young men and young women are told to save themselves for marriage, in practice only women are expected to obey this commandment. For the most part, boys are actively encouraged to engage in extramarital sex, whether as a means of gaining the experience necessary to "satisfy" their future wives, or simply as a way of validating their masculinity.

RESISTANCE TO DOMINANT DISCOURSES

As one might imagine, contradiction leads to acts of resistance. Although these acts are dispersed in time and space, their objective is always the same: to challenge, to confront, to contradict, to question, and in the process to foster new ideas, new principles, new myths, and new forms of symbolism. As Foucault makes clear, just as power relations cut across and through existing structures and institutions, so does resistance, with strategic codification and mobilization that provide the basis for revolutionary action.

Of course, for the most part resistance is not codified in this manner, but is rather amorphous and unfocused, manifesting itself simultaneously in any number of sites and ways. In the paragraphs that follow we provide examples of some of the most common forms that this resistance takes.

One such manifestation involves the deployment of "rational" arguments against hegemonic discourses. These include such statements as "women should be free to work just like men," or "cohabitation amounts to the same thing as marriage." Along similar lines, individuals may seek to modify or reinterpret discursive commandments rather than challenging them directly, as in the case of young people who accept the basic precepts of Christian sexuality while at the same time celebrating the physical pleasure to be derived from the sex act itself. Or, in parallel fashion, one may cite examples of self-styled Christians who accept homosexuality as part of the human condition, basing their view on biblical texts that call for tolerance, rather than those which condemn sodomy as an unacceptable evil. Of course, from here it is but a short jump to what is perhaps the most obvious form of "rational" resistance, namely the formulation of alternative discourses through the development of new religions, new philosophies of life and sex, and new views of the world and its significance.

Still, in making this last point by no means do we wish to suggest that deliberately public acts of resistance are necessarily more effective than those that are implicit or hidden. Indeed, one might even go so far as to argue that individuals' everyday, seemingly innocuous actions do more to disrupt the logic of dominant discourses than do the carefully planned and orchestrated interventions of counterhegemonic social movements.

Examples of such "innocuous" behavior include practices that deviate from discursive norms, such as women who are sexually aggressive, men who are directly involved in the raising of their children, or priests who advocate the use of artificial birth control measures. Of course, some go even further, advocating the creation of support groups for victims of spousal abuse, or the adoption of measures that allow women to take control of their own reproductive health.

Also relevant in this regard are activities that undermine dominant sexual discourses by reappropriating physical space for subversive ends. For example, at the same time that Western societies place strict limits upon where and when men can legitimately express their emotions in public (the soccer pitch being one locale where such expressions are allowed), some have taken it upon themselves to challenge these taboos by crying, kissing, or hugging other men in spaces that have been typed "masculine," such as bars, gyms, and sporting events. Similar resistance is also discernable among individuals who have sex in "illegitimate" locales, such as beaches and school classrooms, or at "inappropriate" times of the day (i.e., during daylight hours). Indeed, time is especially interesting in this regard, given the degree to which it provides the basis for the creation of heterotopic sites on particular days of the year (e.g., Carnival, New Year's Eve), when "alternative" sexualities can be expressed without fear of censure or reprisal.

One might argue that individuals are engaged in resistance when they partake of sexual practices that fall beyond the bounds of the "normal." Although sexual minorities provide what is perhaps the clearest example of such resistance, similar forces are at work among those who seek to redefine sexual intercourse by changing the order of events, or by engaging in alternative forms of penetration.

Finally, resistance may also be expressed in what is *not* said or done. Most notably, this includes individuals who reject the objectification inherent in dominant forms of sexuality by refusing to become implicated in them, for example, by dressing conservatively or devoting themselves to religion or study. Alternatively, fantasy may also become a form of resistance, as in the case of individuals who express their dissatisfaction with the norm by imagining how it would feel to be with different partners, or engage in "deviant" sexual acts.

COMPARTMENTALIZATION OF DISCOURSES

As we have noted above, sexual discourses, along with the power relations with which they are associated, contribute to the production of a sexual culture that is at once fragmented and contradictory. This in turn forces individuals to control and regulate their sexuality in numerous ways, repressing it in some locales (e.g., church, school), while giving it free rein in others (e.g., beaches, discotheques).

As a way of dealing with these widely divergent expectations, the mind compartmentalizes feelings and thoughts pertaining to different forms of sexual expression, causing individuals to become disengaged from themselves and their wider environment.

The Spanish saying "a saint on Sunday and a sinner on weekdays" exemplifies the consequences arising from this type of compartmentalization. Examples are legion: students who speak out in favor of sexual equality during classtime yet harass their female colleagues after hours; men who secretly dress as women; priests who enjoy pornography; "heterosexual" men and women who sleep with individuals of the same sex; young people who indicate that they understand the importance of always wearing a condom, yet refrain from using one with certain partners. In each case, the people involved are able to rationalize their behavior by simply refusing to acknowledge the degree of contradiction inherent within it. Although this may very well help to alleviate individuals' feelings of tension or stress, there are clearly numerous dangers in fencing off parts of one's life in this way, most notably the risk of disarticulating one's actions from their consequences.

Chapter 5

Hegemonic Sexual Discourses

As our research in Villa del Mar and Villa del Sol made clear, both towns are characterized by three dominant sexual discourses, namely those concerning religion, gender, and science. In large measure, their hegemony can be explained by the support they receive from some of the country's key institutions, including the family, the state, the Roman Catholic Church, and the mass media. Given this level of support, one assumes that they are equally hegemonic in other Costa Rican communities, and not merely those which we visited.

In the pages that follow, we will explore the bases of these discourses as they are communicated to, and internalized by, the young people of Villa del Mar and Villa del Sol. Although the issues addressed will be broadly similar in each case, it should be noted that we will be drawing upon slightly different sources of information. While our discussion of gender-based discourses will depend principally upon findings derived from the interviews, our exploration of discourses grounded in religion and science will also make use of relevant textual material, specifically the catechism and literature associated with the fields of sexology and reproductive health.

PRINCIPLES OF RELIGIOUS DISCOURSES

Creation Is Divine and Heterosexuality the Accepted Norm

According to Christian doctrine, God created man, woman, and the world in which we live. Sexuality is seen as part of a divine plan, insight into which can only be gained through study of the Bible and other sacred texts. So what precisely do these texts tell us?

As the catechismal teachings of the Roman Catholic Church make clear, "Man and Woman have been created, which is to say, willed by God: on the one hand, in perfect equality as human persons; on the other, in their respective beings as man and woman" (Conferencia Episcopal Uruguaya, 1992).

Thus, not only did God create man and woman, but he wills them to be together, a sentiment that is given voice repeatedly in biblical writings. For example, in Genesis 2:18, God is reported to have said, "It is not good that man is alone. I will make him a helper that is fit for him" (de Brower, 1975). Needless to say, woman is to be this helper, whose creation provided the basis for the two sexes, "each [made] for the other" (Conferencia Episcopal Uruguaya, 1992).

Seen from this perspective, it is scarcely surprising that sexual identity in general, and heterosexuality in particular, are thought to be directly traceable to God and his divine plan. This is underscored by the Church's official pronouncement on the subject: "everyone, Man and Woman, should acknowledge and accept his sexual identity" (Conferencia Episcopal Uruguaya, 1992). The implications of this statement are twofold. In short, not only does it serve to remind us why Christian discourses in general are so hostile to change (What right do mere mortals have to question God's work?), but it leaves individual priests and others in the Church hierarchy with substantial room to interpret official texts (such as the catechism) according to their own priorities and prejudices.

Significantly, this variability in interpretation was confirmed during the course of the in-depth interviews, with Marianela, a young woman from Villa del Mar, reporting that, in her church, she was told that women should "always be pregnant because they were created from Adam's rib and their mission in life is to have children." Along somewhat different lines, Kenneth and Santiago, youngsters from Villa del Mar, indicated that they believe sexual relations to be reflective of God's work and that, as such, their sanctity must be respected: "If God made them, He must have had a reason."

Only a Fine Line Separates Sexuality from Sin

The Roman Catholic Church defines sin as a "transgression of God's law." Needless to say, the first such transgression was that of

Adam, whose act of biting into an apple from the tree of knowledge resulted in his (and Eve's) ejection from the Garden of Eden, and the tainting of all his descendants until the day of final judgment. Within this frame of analysis human sexuality is deemed part of God's punishment, whereby man and woman's union is subjected to "tensions," and their relations to "desire and domination." Indeed, the only mortal who is believed to have escaped the blemish of original sin is the Virgin Mary, who conceived Christ without recourse to sex (Conferencia Episcopal Uruguaya, 1992).

Thus, as a result of Church teachings, young people in Villa del Mar and Villa del Sol tend to view pleasure in somewhat negative terms, which is not surprising considering the number of times they have been told that "sexual pleasure is morally suspect when pursued for its own sake, in isolation from its procreative and unitive purposes" (Conferencia Episcopal Uruguaya, 1992). Kenneth, for one, emphasized the degree to which Catholics think that "sexuality is terrible . . . all they talk about is sin." This point was also reiterated by Hilda, who feels that the Church expects her to seek "forgiveness for everything . . . even if I fart I'm supposed to ask for forgiveness, forgiveness, forgiveness." The overwhelming majority of interview participants indicated that they had received no sex education from pastors, priests, or other religious officials.

Of course, the fact that members of Roman Catholic religious orders are themselves expected to remain chaste contributes to young people's difficulty in reconciling sexuality with spirituality. Paula, for example, attended a religious school where the nuns were too "embarrassed" to discuss sex and, when asked about it, became "frightened." Similarly, Jorge indicated that he believed that priests' problem with sex resided in the fact that "they had to take a vow of chastity."

Sex Is Morally Debasing

Sex has the power to lead human beings astray and is one of the root causes of moral decay, both at present and in ancient times. Time and time again the story of Sodom and Gomorrah is presented to young people as one of the foremost examples of what happens to those who fall prey to sexual depravation. As focus group participants made clear, catechism lessons are full of warnings concerning the corrupting power of sex and sexuality, with Adam and Eve's fall from grace cited as a case in point.

Needless to say, conservative social groups such as the Christian Family Movement are in full agreement with this view, arguing as it does that sexual "permissiveness" is responsible for the vast bulk of Costa Rica's social problems. Thus, if the country is to rid itself of its current malaise, it is critical that respect for "faithful and fertile love" be instilled in the hearts of all citizens (Movimiento Familiar Cristiano, 1992, p. 26).

As one might imagine, the articulation of sexual practices with the state of the country's well-being is used by priests and other religious officials as a way of discouraging youth from engaging in sex prior to marriage. However, as was made clear during the course of the qualitative interviews, in many cases it has had the opposite effect, with Tatiana arguing that many young people have distanced themselves from religion: "It's become a way of rebelling. Sex is the 'in' thing really. It's like this is the fashionable thing to do now." Meanwhile, Maikol noted that young people have left the Church because of "sex, alcoholism, and drugs," a view confirmed by Jonathan, who felt that sex was an evil thing that makes people "go berserk and do dirty things."

Those Who Have Sex Are Doing the Devil's Work

For Christians, good and evil are forces that wage constant battle with one another on both the physical and spiritual planes. Thus, when a wrongful act is committed, a real figure, embodying pure evil, is invoked as an explanatory device. As the catechism puts it, "Satan . . . and the other demons are fallen angels who have freely refused to serve God and His plan. Their choice against God is definitive. They try to associate Man in their revolt against God" (Conferencia Episcopal Uruguaya, 1992).

In the context of the interviews, it is clear that many participants have internalized this particular belief. For example, Tatiana explained her failure to attend Mass for three months by saying that "I've got a little devil in me." Meanwhile, Maikol reported that his mother regularly tells him to go to church to "get the devil out" of him.

Sex is thought to be one of Satan's favorite tools in inducing men and women to become sinful and perverted. This in turn explains why the young people interviewed tended to describe their sexual peccadillos as instances when "the devil got inside of them." In the face of the threat posed by such temptation, the Church makes use of its own battery of magic-religious weapons, including confession, prayer, and atonement.

Marriage Is a Means of Avoiding Sins of the Flesh

Given the tendency within Christian circles to associate unbridled sexuality with the devil, what avenues are open to believers who wish to express their sexual identity in ways that are consistent with Church doctrine? Certainly, they will find little solace in the writings of the early Church fathers. Paul, for example, believed that abstinence was the only path to a spiritual life; marriage came in a poor second in his estimation. A similar position was espoused by Clement of Alexandria, who saw sexual relations as a "slight epilepsy, an incurable disease . . . that is why it's harmful: Man is insane in the frenzy of coitus" (Bullough, 1976, p. 198).

However, despite the strongly negative attitude of the early Church, over time its position became increasingly pragmatic, with marital intercourse eventually being accepted as a legitimate expression of human sexuality. Interestingly, many of the interview and focus group participants appear to share the Church's views on the sanctity of marriage, given the extent to which they voiced disapproval of extramarital sex. While some suggested that the Church's prohibition of such behavior was fair because "it's God's will," others simply made reference to their priest's condemnation of the practice.

The Purpose of Marriage Is Union and Procreation

At the same time that it affirms the sacredness of marriage in the eyes of God, the catechism goes on to ground marriage's usefulness in its capacity to engender life itself. Needless to say, in doing so it condemns all sexual activities that are not oriented toward reproduction, arguing that "sexual pleasure . . . sought outside of the sexual relationship which is demanded by the moral order" runs counter to God's will (Conferencia Episcopal Uruguaya, 1992).

As one might imagine, the young people who participated in this study are very familiar with the Church's position on the purpose of marriage, arguing frequently during the course of the in-depth interviews that sex should serve to "complement," "unite," "attract," and "create love" among men and women, and that its underlying raison d'être was to allow couples to "have children and establish a family."

Virginity Is a Requirement for Marriage

Christianity places great stock in virginity. Everyone who is baptized in a Roman Catholic Church is called upon to follow Christ's example and lead a chaste life, in accordance with their status and situation. Thus, while the clergy take a vow of celibacy and married couples one of fidelity, fiancés are expected to "reserve for marriage the expressions of affection that belong to married love" (Conferencia Episcopal Uruguaya, 1992).

However, the requirement that one be a virgin on the day of one's marriage is more rigorously enforced for women than it is for men. This is underscored by the interview responses of men such as David, who, despite being gay and a prostitute, said that he would never marry a woman "who isn't dressed in white." This is not to say that men are completely exempt from these pressures themselves. As Jorge put it, both women *and* men should remain celibate before marriage, inasmuch as one "should give all of oneself to the person one marries."

Masturbation Corrupts

According to the tenets of the Jewish religion, it is a grave sin to waste one's semen, recalling as it does Onan's decision to spill his seed in the desert, rather than impregnate his brother's widow as Levitical law required (Deuteronomy 25:6). Although his crime consisted essentially of disobeying his father and disregarding traditional Levitical requirements, scrupulous biblical scholars have since argued that the condemnation of Onan encompasses a proscription of all forms of semen emission that are nonprocreative in orientation.

As one might imagine, it is on the basis of this interpretation that masturbation, together with oral sex and contraceptive use, are considered serious offenses in the eyes of the Church hierarchy and the Roman Catholic catechism, with the latter proclaiming that "the deliberate use of the sexual faculty, for whatever reason, outside of marriage is essentially contrary to its purpose" (par. 2352). Moreover, it goes on to argue that "both the Magisterium of the Church . . . and the moral sense of the faithful have been in no doubt and have firmly maintained that masturbation is an intrinsically and gravely disordered action" (par. 2352).

To a large extent, interview participants appear to have internalized this perspective, with Gisella indicating that she had been taught that masturbation "goes against Christian values." As for Jorge, he argued that the practice should be avoided because "one is not giving love to anyone," while Susan asserted that it is sinful, and thus should simply not be done.

All Thoughts of Fornication Should Be Banished from One's Mind

According to the catechism, not only does fornication entail "carnal union between an unmarried man and an unmarried woman" (par. 2353), but it is "gravely contrary to the dignity of persons and of human sexuality which is naturally ordered to the good of spouses and the generation and education of children" (par. 2353).

Given this view, it is not particularly surprising that so many of the study participants felt that desire was sinful. Yet, even as they expressed this sentiment, they did go on to make a distinction between appropriate and inappropriate objects of desire. According to Leidy, "desire is sinful if one is not married." However, as Alexandria put it, so long as the woman whom a man is undressing with his eyes is his wife, "it's not a sin."

Prostitution Is a Social Scourge

In the eyes of Church leaders, prostitution is an assault upon the dignity of the prostitute's body, to the extent that he or she is reduced to an object of sexual pleasure. Meanwhile, the buyer of sex sins gravely by being unchaste and by defiling his (or her) body (Conferencia Episcopal Uruguaya, 1992).

Although it was evident in the group sessions and interviews that young people agree with the Church on the sinfulness of prostitution, many went on to temper their condemnation by suggesting that some individuals are driven to the sex trade by factors beyond their control, such as "the need to feed their children," "lack of education," "helplessness," or "being abandoned by her man."

Using Pornography Is a Serious Offense

A similarly negative attitude pervades the Church's views on pornography. As the catechism makes clear, pornography involves the removal of "sexual acts from the intimacy of partners in order to display them deliberately to third parties. It is an offense to chastity because it perverts the conjugal act . . . it does grave injury to the dignity of those who participate in it" (par. 2354).

A significant number of participants agreed that watching pornographic films was sinful, explaining their refusal to watch them by saying they wanted "to avoid sin," "to respect their religion," or "to avoid divine punishment."

Homosexuality Is Unnatural

Defining homosexuality as "relations between men or women who experience an exclusive or predominant sexual attraction toward persons of the same sex" (par. 2357) the Roman Catholic catechism goes on to make the following claims about it: homosexuality has taken a great variety of forms through the centuries . . . Its psychological genesis remains largely unexplained. Basing itself on Sacred Scripture . . . (Genesis 19:1-29; Romans 1:1-29; I Corinthians 6:9; I Timothy 1:10), "tradition has always declared that homosexual acts are intrinsically disordered. They are contrary to the natural law. They are an affront to the sexual act to the gift of life. They do not proceed from genuine affective or sexual complementarity. Under no circumstances can they be approved" (par. 2357).

During the course of the in-depth interviews, a number of young people came forward to express their disdain for homosexuality.

Kenneth, for example, indicated that "God didn't make the penis and balls to go into the anus, which is for getting rid of bodily waste." Alexandra agreed, saying that "God made man and woman to complement each other." Even David, who is himself gay, said that "homosexuality should not exist on earth . . . God made man and woman to be together and I chose the wrong path."

Adultery Is a Serious Offense

The Roman Catholic Church takes adultery very seriously, if religious writings and sacred texts are any guide. According to Matthew 5:27-28, Christ condemned all forms of adultery, even that of mere desire. Along similar lines, the sixth commandment forbids adultery absolutely (cf. Matthew 5:27-28, 32 and 19:6; Mark 10:11; I Corinthians 6:9-10), while the prophets denounced the practice as akin to the sin of idolatry" (Conferencia Episcopal Uruguaya, 1992).

For the most part, young people share this view, and deem adultery to be a serious offense against the sanctity of marriage. To cite but two examples, Susana argued that it is "one of the worst calamities facing religion," while Carlos saw its prevalence as "proof of the decline in religious values."

Divorce Is Contrary to Divine Law

As Church writings make clear, "the Lord Jesus insisted that the Creator's original intention was for marriage to be indissoluble" (cf. Matthew 5:31-32; Mark 10:9; Leviticus 16:18; I Corinthians 7:10-11). This in turn has led the framers of the catechism to argue that no human power other than death can legitimately break up a ratified and consummated marriage among individuals who have been baptized (par. 2382).

Needless to say, young people showed themselves to be very familiar with the Church's prohibition of divorce. Tatiana, for one, argued that "It does not matter how many divorce papers a couple gets; as far as the Church is concerned they're still married." As for Maria, she felt that, since the institution of marriage is derived ultimately from God, couples should take to heart the saying "Till death do us part."

Children Should Not Be Avoided

As for matters of family planning, the catechism is quite explicit in its condemnation of "morally unacceptable means" of preventing pregnancy, such as sterilization and the use of oral contraceptives (par. 2399). Interview and focus group participants were clearly well versed in current debates on the subject, with Vanessa indicating that she knew that the Church was against family planning "because having children is a privilege that one should not be deprived of." Meanwhile, both Jorge and Guillermo are familiar with the conflict between Church and state over the distribution of sex education material in schools, and know that the Roman Catholic hierarchy "opposes condoms and other methods of family planning."

Abortion Is Murder

In the eyes of the Roman Catholic Church, "human life must be respected and protected absolutely from the moment of conception. From the first moment of his existence, a human being must be recognized as having the rights of a person, among which is the inviolable right of every innocent being to life (cf. CDF, Donum Vitae, 1, 1) Since the first century, the Church has affirmed the moral evil of every produced abortion. This teaching has not changed and remains unchangeable" (Conferencia Episcopal Uruguaya, 1992).

Clearly, most of the young people interviewed were equally opposed to abortion in all of its forms. In short, abortion and murder were deemed to be one and the same, with the only exception being cases where the mother's life was in danger. As Maria put it, "Abortion should only be considered if the mother risks dying herself, since the child is unborn and what could a child do without its mother?"

PRINCIPLES OF GENDER DISCOURSES

In Costa Rica, religious discourses are complemented by those of gender. Although one might argue that the latter's roots are considerably more diverse than those of the former, given the degree to which misogyny and sex-based inequity are common strands throughout the Western world, it is clear that the two discourses reinforce each other in reproducing a particular understanding of human sexuality.

Sexual Roles Are Determined by Organs, Instinct, and Hormones

Within this frame of reference, masculinity and femininity are determined by the presence or absence of a penis. This is confirmed by Jonathan, who asserted during the course of our interview with him, "I am masculine because I have a penis, let's say women are feminine because they have a vagina." Being in possession of a penis is thought to render one more aggressive and sex-driven. Thus, not only did Danny and Juan argue that they were "stronger" because of their penises, but Susana indicated that she thought women were weaker due to the presence of female hormones in their bodies.

Indeed, the importance of hormones cannot be understated in this regard, given the significance attributed to them by study participants. All in all, the vast majority of young people interviewed indicated that they thought hormones, along with instinct and sexual organs, were key determinants of masculine and feminine behavior.

Sex Roles Are Grounded in Biology

In light of the discussion above, it is not particularly surprising that most of the research participants (whether male or female) believed that men, by virtue of their sex, were naturally strong, aggressive, assertive, and hardworking, whereas women were submissive, passive, vain, and delicate. In Katia's words, "It's simply natural that this is the case."

Role Determines Function

Along similar lines, many of the young people involved in the study indicated that women's natural environment is the home, while that of men is the (wage-paying) workplace and the street. In the focus group session, mention was often made of the importance of girls getting married in order to bear and raise children, and of men going to work to support their families. Several female participants stated that women's nurturing skills were grounded in biology, with Rosangela and Wendy in particular saying that girls' fondness for dolls was innate, the product of menstruation, which serves to render them more sensitive and care-oriented.

Man/Woman, Active/Passive

In the minds of most study participants, men are active by nature whereas women are passive, with activity and passivity measured according to one's ability to penetrate others. Thus, since it is only men who possess a penetrative sexual organ, not only does it follow (in the peculiar logic of dominant gender discourses) that men should be more sexually active than women, but that it is better to penetrate than to be penetrated.

This is underscored by the views expressed by Kenneth, who believes that women who agree to have sex with him are "sluts" and that they deserve to be abandoned afterward. As he puts it:

> The first week I hug her, the following week I touch her breasts, the week after that I'm getting inside her, and by the following week she's already sleeping with me. In one month the work's all done. It's like arm wrestling—if she's tough it's more fun because it's more of a challenge.

The superior value attributed to penetration is reflected in the language used to describe men and women's sexual organs. During the in-depth interviews, the penis was typically depicted as a powerful and violent weapon: pistol, rifle, bat, bar, stick, machine gun, club, and nail were only some of the words used in this regard. By contrast, the vagina was generally portrayed in terms suggestive of inferiority and passivity: for example, hole, frog, monkey, pit, crater, or crack.

Penetrated Women Are Sluts Unless They Are Married

During the course of our interview with him, Kenneth described himself as a "male prostitute," since he loves nothing more than going to bed with women. However, while thinking nothing of this, he went on to say that a woman who did the same would be thought a "slut" by everyone. To illustrate this point he related an anecdote:

> [A] friend pretended to be drunk, and he started to get all lovey-dovey with a girl. They started to make love, even though she was saying no, and then finally he stuck it in her and she ended up liking it. Later on, when he was telling me about it, he said, "That bitch, what a phoney, she said no, it's disgusting and all that, and then suddenly she's into it."

Indeed, even women refer to other women who have lost their virginity as "whores" and "sluts." Susana, for one, argued that a woman should only give herself to her husband; if she has sex with her fiancé, she becomes worthless.

Men Who Are Sexually Active Are Manly and Admired

According to Kenneth, being a real man entails having sex as much as possible: "Yeah, I've fucked women in the street, on the beach, and at home, though if it's at home I'm always careful to make sure that my mother doesn't walk in." Meanwhile, Carlos indicated that being manly means being willing to "eat out any woman's cunt or asshole." He admitted that "feeling girls up" was his favorite pastime, and that he loves to get together with his friends to talk about recent sexual exploits.

Not only did most of the other male participants voice broadly similar points of view, but many of the young women interviewed agreed that men should be more knowledgeable about sex, with several indicating that they would find it exceedingly difficult to ask a man out or initiate sexual activity. For these participants, the man should play the role of "guide" and "teacher" during the course of their sexual encounter.

Women Should Never Act Suggestively or Provocatively Toward Men

Among the male research participants, it was widely argued that women who act suggestively in the company of men run the risk of being raped. As Kenneth put it, "Sometimes the eyes tell you—they say no, but their eyes and their body language say yes. In cases like that, it's okay to use force." Female participants, including Maria, indicated that women must be very careful in how they present themselves, and that they must never go into the street and do things which might serve to "provoke men."

PRINCIPLES OF SCIENTIFIC DISCOURSES

With the development of modern psychiatry in the nineteenth century, a new discourse began to take shape, one that was particularly useful to the state as a means of regulating and controlling the social (and sexual) lives of citizens. Internalized and propagated by such groups as psychiatrists, sexologists, physicians, demographers, sociologists, lawyers, economists, and criminologists, the tenets of scientific discourse flew squarely in the face of the assumptions built into religious discourses, and frequently those of gender discourses as well.

Sexual Health Should Be a State Priority

From the moment that economists, demographers, and sociologists adopted the position that population was a key factor in either facilitating or hindering development, public health, the practice of birth control, and the spread of STDs took on growing importance in the calculations of state managers.

Because of this, the state began increasingly to intervene in areas touching upon citizens' biological reproduction and sexual practices. In countries where labor power was in short supply, emphasis was placed upon encouraging families to have more children. Conversely, in overpopulated regions, contraceptive use, sterilization, and deferral of first pregnancy were encouraged. Meanwhile, at a personal level, the belief that resource availability should determine family size and that every couple has the right to practice birth control gained wider and wider currency. In the context of the present study, this is seen in Hilda's repetition of such advertising slogans as "Have only the number of children you can afford to make happy," and in Jorge's comment that "These days you can't make the mistake of having too many children. You have to use the methods available."

Along somewhat different lines, the spread of HIV/AIDS in Costa Rica, with its tendency to strike down those who are in the prime of their economically productive years, has induced the government to become a keen proponent of both condom use and AIDS awareness among the population at large. To a significant degree, these efforts appear to be bearing fruit, given study participants' knowledge of risk factors, and statements by individuals such as José that "there's no question that you have to use a glove [condom] when you're having sex, even though it's uncomfortable."

Furthermore, at the same time that experts (psychiatrists, psychologists, and others) have taken it upon themselves to determine the bounds between "normal" and "abnormal" sexuality (with the latter generally including all that is not heterosexual in orientation), the state has drawn upon this knowledge in its own efforts to discourage "abnormal" sexual practices. As the in-depth interviews make clear, it has been quite successful in promoting its views in this area, with participants such as Manuel arguing that "People who fuck children, rapists, faggots, whores, and drug-addicts should all be jailed."

Sexual Orientation/Identity Arises Through "Internal" Processes of Psychological Development

People are thought to acquire their sexual orientation and gender identity through the interplay of biological and psychological processes. It should be noted that Freudian views on the close relationship between parent-child interactions and sexual orientation are particularly prevalent in Costa Rica.

In this way, "normal" sexual development is thought to lead to heterosexuality, to the degree that relations between men and women are a necessary prerequisite for the reproduction of the species. Should something occur to thwart this process, abnormal or "deviant" sexuality is the result. In the context of the interviews, this belief manifested itself often, as is seen in the following statement by Alexandro: "Homosexuality is an illness that can be cured, if they want to."

Sex Is Natural and Produces Pleasure

Freud (1917) argues that sexuality is mostly about pleasure; procreation is merely an accidental result. Given this perspective, individuals' repression of sexual desire exacts a price, most notably in the area of mental health. Thus, to the extent that state and parastate agents have internalized this understanding, sex is no longer viewed in moral or religious terms, but is seen instead as a means of encouraging or discouraging demographic growth.

Women and Men Have Similar Sex Drives

In sharp contrast to the gender-based discourses outlined above, sexology is grounded in the view that, despite the existence of certain physiological differences, in no way can one distinguish men and women on the basis of their sex drive or capacity to experience sexual pleasure. Given this perspective, the purpose of marriage ceases to be merely that of union and procreation, as the dictates of Christianity demand, but becomes centered around *pleasure* as well. Evidence suggests that at least some of the study participants have internalized this view, as seen in Lucrecia's assertion that "men and women should enjoy sex."

Some Techniques Must Be Learned for Sex to Be Satisfying

Sexologists argue that both men and women have rights as well as obligations in sexual intercourse. There should be more to sex than penetration and male orgasm. Rather, the sex act should be accompanied by other forms of stimulation, with the ultimate goal being the satisfaction of *both* partners' needs and desires.

As one might imagine, this in turn has served to widen the field of "legitimate" sexual practices. No longer is it considered deviant to engage in oral sex or masturbation. As Frederico put it, "Jacking off is normal. We all do it at one time or another, and we haven't gone mad as they said we would."

Communication Is an Essential Ingredient of Good Sex

Given this heightened emphasis upon satisfying one's partner's desires, it is vital that couples be able to speak frankly to one another, if only to say what gives them pleasure and what does not. Thus, both sexologists and psychologists have come to stress the importance of verbal communication as a way of resolving sexual problems.

Being Able to Satisfy One's Partner Is Important; Being a Virgin Is Not

Couples who remain celibate until marriage run the risk of being sexually incompatible. Thus, sexologists will often recommend pre-marital experimentation, particularly if there is strong evidence of love between the individuals involved. Needless to say, virginity has no place within this frame of reference. Although one might argue that many Costa Rican men continue to expect their wives to have no prior sexual experience, statements made by research participants suggest that change is afoot in this area. Jorge, for example, while indicating that he would prefer to marry someone who is a virgin, went on to say that "We all lose our virginity at some point and if she [i.e., his future wife] lost it with someone else, I would still marry her, because that's why I would want to get married, because I love her."

Lack of Sexual Satisfaction Is One Cause of Divorce

Sexologists and psychologists argue that marriages can fail for many reasons, of which one is sexual incompatibility: couples may not like the same things, their respective sex drives may differ, and so on. In these cases, if communication and/or therapy does not resolve the underlying problems, divorce may be a necessary and advisable course of action. As one might imagine, this perspective stands in direct opposition to the tenets of religious discourse, which considers divorce to be an affront to God's will.

Chapter 6

Assimilation of Religious Discourses

Although Christ had relatively little to say about sex during his own lifetime, he made it quite clear that he was opposed to divorce, not least because of his concern for women abandoned in this way. In an oft-cited passage from Matthew 19:12, he is reported to have offered praise for "male eunuchs who made themselves so to serve the Kingdom of Heaven" (de Brower, 1975). While some early Christians took this statement to mean that God requires abstinence from his followers, others who were more literal in their interpretation went so far as to castrate themselves. Although Origen, who died ca. 254 A.D., was perhaps the most notable example of this latter stream of thought, by the fourth century the Church hierarchy had prohibited all acts of genital self-mutilation (Bullough, 1976).

If definitive statements by Christ on the subject of sexuality were most notable by their absence, Paul more than made up for this silence by engaging in detailed interpretations of Christ's words. While stressing that celibacy is always the best course of action for Christians wishing to lead a spiritual life, he acknowledged that marriage is an acceptable (if inferior) alternative for those who are tempted by the pleasures of the flesh.

As for his views on women, Paul was adamant that they were the principal source of sexual temptation, citing Adam and Eve's fall from grace as evidence in support of this conclusion. It was this belief that led him to call for women's subordination at the hands of their husbands or fathers, so that their powers of seduction might not lead other men astray. Of course, among the sins they might induce men to commit, few were as serious as extramarital sex. The New Testament is exceedingly clear on this point: adultery, fornication, sodomy, and masturbation were absolutely and completely forbidden.

Still, it must be acknowledged that the early Church's hostility toward sex did not develop in a social vacuum. The Near East was rife with ascetic religious sects in the early centuries of the Christian era, many of which were in direct competition with Christianity for followers, thereby forcing Christianity to adopt many of its rivals' ideas in a bid to make itself more marketable.

Two sects that were particularly influential in this regard were Gnosticism and Manichaeism. Although the former was denounced by Clement of Alexandria in the second century, its abhorrence of the material world in general, and temptations of the flesh in particular, had already proved influential among leading Christian scholars of the time, of which Justin Martyr is the most notable example. These ascetic tendencies were reinforced in turn by the co-option of Manichaeist doctrine by St. Augustine, among others. Briefly, Manichaeism posited a universe divided into kingdoms of light and darkness, with human beings poised between the two, their bodies the product of darkness, yet in possession of souls that were derived from the kingdom of light. Thus, each individual must endeavor to free his or her soul from its bodily shackles by abstaining from sex, eating a diet free of meat, and so on. Although Augustine was once a follower of Manes himself, his inability to control his own bodily desires had led him to reject Manichaeism in favor of Christianity, though he held onto his dim view of all things related to human sexuality, with the single exception being sex for the sake of procreation. Needless to say, his ideas have since proven to be extremely influential in the development of Church doctrine on matters touching upon sex and reproduction.

THE COSTA RICAN CONTEXT

During the early phase of Spanish colonial expansion into the Americas, a shortage of labor combined with the relative weakness of social control mechanisms contributed to something of a relaxation in Christian sexual norms, particularly in regions (e.g., Costa Rica) that were far removed from the power centers of the time.

Thus, even as the Roman Catholic hierarchy in colonial San José condemned divorce and fornication, it was pragmatic enough to recognize its own powerlessness to enforce these edicts, along with the agricultural sector's desperate need for laborers. In the face of these contradictions, the Church became increasingly concerned with form rather than substance, while turning a blind eye to the burgeoning population of "illegitimate" children.

A similar outlook characterized the Catholic Church's views on the conversion of indigenous peoples. According to Ricardo Blanco, a priest who has carried out an extensive examination of the Costa Rican Church's historical development, evangelization of the native population was never a priority for the Spanish colonialists. Quite simply, the Spanish believed that real conversion to Christianity was not feasible due to the poor intellectual capacities of indigenous people, together with the great differences that were thought to exist between Christianity and native religions (Blanco, 1967).

As for Church leaders' attitude toward the Spanish settlers, their two principal concerns revolved around ensuring that the population remained at least nominally Catholic on the one hand (i.e., that they partook of the principal sacraments), and the advancement of their own political agenda on the other. As one might imagine, the latter point is an important one, underlining as it does the fact that the Church was closely allied to the Costa Rican state structure from its very inception.

This cozy arrangement would remain largely unquestioned until the 1960s, when liberation theology began to make inroads among segments of the Costa Rican priesthood. At the very moment that rank-and-file members of the clergy became increasingly vocal in their criticism of conservative Church leaders, the latter were faced with a threat from an entirely new direction: Protestant missionaries from North America eager to gain converts among the country's low and middle classes. The missionaries' efforts in this regard have been hugely successful, leading to a 300 percent increase in Evangelical Church membership over the course of the past three decades. Today, as much as 15 percent of the country's population self-identifies as Protestant.

Drawing inspiration from Scripture, fundamentalist churches in Costa Rica have sought to reenergize Christianity by championing the (supposed) values and mores of the early Church. In matters of sex and sexuality, this entails an emphasis upon abstinence before marriage, and condemnation of family planning, abortion, and all sexual practices that are not heterosexual in orientation. Moreover, it should be noted as well that these churches have joined the Roman Catholic hierarchy in staunchly opposing sex education in the public school system, while promoting their own, religiously based educational programs instead.

Evidence of contradiction within dominant religious discourses serves to promote change in the way that youth think and act. State policy and gender and class relations, along with the effects of epidemics such as AIDS, are among the forces that might be influential in this regard, to the degree that they induce young people to reinterpret or challenge "orthodox" principles and demands. In the paragraphs that follow, we examine the role of gender in shaping discourse, paying particular attention to the different ways in which men and women assimilate and modify the dictates of religion.

FEMALE RELIGIOUS DISCOURSES

By now it should be obvious that discourses are never able to impose themselves with absolute authority. Thus, despite the fact that ethnographic observation has shown women in Costa Rica to be more likely than men to participate in religious activities, it does not necessarily follow that they are faithful adherents to Church doctrine. As will be made clear in the discussion below, some precepts are accepted, while others are not.

Our interviews with female participants underscored the degree to which women's religious orientation is shaped through the interplay of Church doctrine with their own interpersonal relations. In effect, this means that women's willingness to believe in the divine origin of religious edicts (e.g., prohibition of divorce) does not prevent them from discarding them should these edicts endanger of the stability of their personal lives. In cases such as these, the offending precept is relegated to the status of exception, while those injunctions which have no bearing on close friends or family members are more readily accepted.

With regard to sexuality in particular, the young women interviewed do not believe that it is simply a means of procreation (the Church's position), but see it instead as a way of expressing affection within a caring, loving relationship. This is confirmed by the comments of participants such as Hilda, who indicated that sex is a "way of uniting with another person." Needless to say, it is but a short step from this perspective to the view that loving sex, even outside of marriage, is not a sin. As Adriana put it, "If some day I really love somebody and want to have intercourse with him, so what, I will!"

Significantly, even in cases where female participants do support the Catholic Church's prohibition of extramarital sex, this generally has less to do with religious conviction than with individuals' concern over what might occur should they engage in such activity. Thus, for example, Paula has decided to remain celibate before marriage "because of the consequences of being a single mother."

The issue of divorce draws out an analogous set of responses among the young women who participated in the study. If relations between husband and wife are sufficiently destructive, and if the children are being negatively affected, most would be willing to consider divorce as a way out of an impossible situation. Thus, while Susana and Leidy indicated that it was justified in cases of adultery, violence, and mistreatment, Marianela stated quite simply, "If the couple's unhappy, they should do it." Hilda is equally pragmatic, saying "If there's no way to sort things out, then what else is there to do?"

Prostitution receives similar treatment at the hands of the women interviewed. Paula argued that it should not be seen as sin when "the mother does it to save her children." Yahaira agrees, drawing a distinction between cases where it is driven by necessity as opposed to pleasure.

Female participants become even less accepting of Church doctrine when it directly affects their independence and personal autonomy. Thus, despite the fact that women are routinely exhorted by priests, pastors, and religious texts to act submissively toward the men in their lives, most of the women interviewed rejected these demands out of hand. In Hilda's words, the expectation that a woman should bow down to her man is simply "not realistic." In a similar vein, Paula feels that "There's a lot of hypocrisy in the Church and that you should be able to make your own decisions."

As for the issue of homosexuality, many were quite negative in their assessment of it, though not, it should be added, because of Church views on the matter. Some said that they were turned off because it was "disgusting" and "dirty," while others thought that it went against the natural scheme of things. For instance, Paula indicated that she does not understand how people can alter the function of sexual organs which are meant to be complementary. In another example, Maria stated that she was opposed to homosexuality because it deprives women of potential mates: "There are gay men who are so good-looking and that's just a waste."

However, it is important to note that women's perspectives change once they become personally acquainted with an individual who is gay or lesbian. Gisella, for one, defends homosexuality because she has a cousin who is gay, and is good friends with his partner as well. As she put it, "No one has the right to meddle in his life." A similar point of view was expressed by Yahaira, who said that she knows several gay men, and "they're all good guys."

Finally, it should be emphasized that young women are also willing to oppose Church doctrine when it places their health or well-being at risk. In short, most of the female participants said that they were entirely willing to use contraceptives and condoms, both to avoid unwanted pregnancies and to minimize the risk of acquiring an STD. Even Susana, who describes herself as fundamentalist on religious matters, indicated that she has no qualms about using prophylactics to ensure that she has no more children than she is able to support.

MALE RELIGIOUS DISCOURSES

As was underscored during the course of the interview and focus group sessions, young men tend to be less devout and less preoccupied with interpersonal relations than their female counterparts. It was also made clear to us that their understanding of what is morally right and wrong is grounded less in the omnipotence of God than in their own sense of order and logic. In this way, young men are most likely to obey religious interdictions that make sense to them on an intellectual level, while those that do not are transgressed with impunity or else simply ignored.

Masturbation is a case in point. Most male participants stated that they had no idea why it was deemed sinful, seeing it as a normal part of their sexual development. As one interviewee put it, "Even priests masturbate to diminish their desire for women." Significantly, even in the limited number of cases where individuals did express opposition to masturbation, they did so in nonreligious terms. For example, Jorge argued that it was a pointless exercise: "You are not giving love to anybody; it's just imaginary."

Analogously, young men's willingness to accept the Church's interdiction against homosexuality is to a large extent based upon their view that this is a "logical" position to take. Arguing that men and women's sexual anatomy is "complementary," most felt that any attempt to engage in alternative forms of sexual practice (such as anal intercourse) must necessarily be a violation of God's will. In Juan's words, gays and lesbians "should come to terms with the way God made them, the sex God made them." Discovering that a friend of his was gay did nothing to alter Juan's perspective; he simply broke off the friendship. Needless to say, this stands in sharp contrast to women in a similar situation, who are generally far more accepting of homosexuality among friends and family members.

As for the question of nonprocreative or extramarital sex, the majority of young men interviewed were far less willing than the Roman Catholic Church to condemn such practices out of hand. Quite simply, most felt that since sex is pleasurable and "natural" it is only right that men should be able to enjoy it, regardless of whether they are married or not. To cite José, "If you run into a chick somewhere, why should you abstain? No way!" However, by the same token it must be acknowledged that several participants felt it made sense to remain celibate prior to marriage. Reasons ranged from the importance of testing one's loyalty to one's partner, to individuals' inability to support children born out of wedlock.

Even so, almost all of the young men who participated in the study disagreed with the Roman Catholic position on divorce and family planning, though once again their views tended to be grounded in logic rather than religious conviction. With regard to divorce in particular, most shared Guillermo's opinion that "the Church has become too strict and puritanical," arguing that, in cases where "partners don't love each other" or "can't get along," divorce is acceptable and cannot be considered a sin. In Danny's words, "It's better for them to stop living together and fooling themselves—otherwise marriage becomes a farce."

There was widespread consensus among participants that condom use and family planning are reasonable measures in the face of present-day realities, which include the risk of contracting HIV/ AIDS and the lack of sufficient resources to care for a large number of children. Indeed, several went so far as to repeat an advertising slogan used by Profamilia, a private company that markets contraceptives in Costa Rica: "Have only the number of children you can afford to make happy."

Finally, with respect to prostitution, it should be noted that the majority of young men interviewed indicated that they were opposed to it. Among the reasons cited were the sense.that it was preposterous to pay for sex, and the belief that most prostitutes could engage in other forms of work if they so wished. To quote Aaron, "Sex is about love rather than money; there are other jobs that don't take away from a woman's dignity." However, like their female counterparts, the men were sensitive enough to realize that there are situations in which prostitution becomes unavoidable, such as the need to meet basic living expenses or support children. As Alan put it, "If a woman's doing it to buy food, it's not a sin."

COMMUNITY RELIGIOUS DISCOURSES

In previous chapters, we have argued that social class plays a significant role in influencing processes of discourse internalization and development. This claim is borne out when we turn our attention to religious discourses in Villa del Mar and Villa del Sol. While the middle-class population of the latter community tends to see religion as dynamic and adaptable in the face of new circumstances, for the relatively poor inhabitants of Villa del Mar not only is the Church more important in their day-to-day lives, but religious belief is much less flexible. That is, it is expected that religion will confront and challenge new realities, rather than adapting to them.

Thus, it is not particularly surprising to learn that religion has lost much of its importance for Villa del Sol's young people. Interview participants felt that it was no longer necessary; that it was akin to idol worship or, in one case, that it should be rejected because it was imposed by Spanish colonizers. As one might imagine, the relative sophistication of the arguments put forth in this regard are closely related to the participants' privileged socioeconomic status. Most have stayed in school far longer than their counterparts in Villa del Mar, and as such have been exposed to information about other religions or alternative perspectives on the Spanish conquest and the imposition of Christianity in the Americas.

Despite the fact that most households in Villa del Sol are characterized by two parents living under the same roof with their children (in other words, the ideal "Christian" family), the young people from this community who participated in the study were generally quite skeptical of the Church's expectations in the area of premarital sex and contraceptive use.

With regard to premarital sex in particular, several participants said that it was "impossible" to remain celibate prior to marriage. Of course, it hardly needs to be emphasized that Villa del Sol youth tend to get married much later in life than those in Villa del Mar, as most of them go on to some form of postsecondary education following the completion of high school. For this reason, long-term celibacy as demanded by the Church is not considered feasible. Kenneth, for one, argues that although abstention is a worthy aim in principle, "It doesn't happen that way in real life, since most people have had sex by the time they're seventeen." Along similar lines, both Gisella and Adriana felt that it was up to each person to decide whether or not to have sex before marriage. As Adriana put it, "It's my choice, not the Church's."

Several young people commented that they had forsaken Christianity precisely because of the emphasis placed upon chastity and virginity. For example, Hilda said that she resents the Catholic Church for its opposition to premarital sex and wishes that it was "more understanding." Gianina, meanwhile, criticized the Church for its refusal to countenance sex education in schools, and longs for the day when mass will be more "fun" and sex will be judged less harshly. Others' attacks were more general in scope, with Paula commenting upon priests' negative attitude toward young people, and José exclaiming that he is sickened by all the "lies" he is told in church.

In Villa del Mar, by contrast, young people look upon Christianity in far more favorable terms. Although the reasons for this are undoubtedly complex, one factor certainly is the preponderance of singe-parent families. In a community where stable marriages are the exception rather than the rule, children and adolescents have every reason to be staunch defenders of the Church's position on divorce and the sanctity of marriage.

Even though there are some young people in Villa del Mar who have rejected the values and dictates of Christianity, most are fervent supporters of them. For instance, Juan said that "Church is an interesting and good place to go," a statement reiterated by Yahaira: "I'm the one who gets up at seven in the morning to do the housework in order to go to Mass. I've always liked it; I like everything they say." Guillermo, who is not a devout Christian, stated that religion is "very important," and provides a means of escaping from the troubles he faces in his everyday life.

This last point is an important one, highlighting as it does the fact that many in Villa del Mar turn to Christianity because they expect it to be able to solve their problems, whether it be a family break-up or the threat posed by poverty, drugs, or alcohol. This expectation is evident in the words of participants. Rosangela, for one, stressed the importance of abstaining from sex before marriage, and said that she often tells her recently divorced sister "to go to church to learn what it was that she did wrong." Juan indicated that he believes "religion to be important because it keeps young people away from vices." Finally, Yahaira, who is single and lives with her parents, said that she respects the Church for "making people stay together in order to save marriages."

Many interview participants in Villa del Mar placed particular emphasis upon the importance of obeying the Church's rules on fornication. Indeed, for some, being able to dress in white at their wedding was one of the most appealing aspects of Christian ritual. In short, while women tended to see virginity as a way of guaranteeing a good marriage in the future, men considered it a useful gauge of their future wife's moral character.

Substance abuse and prostitution are other issues that young people living in Villa del Mar hope will be resolved through faith in God. Several participants indicated that they thought religion was capable of helping drug abusers and prostitutes to make the right choices. In the words of Isidro, "The greatest benefit the Church has to offer is that it makes people abandon drugs." Of course, it need hardly be added that religion actually has to be successful in dealing with these problems if it is to keep young people's respect. However, evidence suggests that this success is not always forthcoming, with several participants expressing disappointment at the reluctance of many priests and ministers to speak frankly about issues that concern them, such as sex and substance abuse.

FUNDAMENTALIST RELIGIOUS DISCOURSES

In the preceding pages, we have endeavored to highlight some of the ways in which sexual discourses can be transformed by socio-economic status, changing gender ideology, and technological innovation. However, even as one acknowledges the degree to which these developments have undermined traditional views of sex and sexuality in Costa Rica, it is clear that not everyone has embraced these new values with open arms.

Religious fundamentalists in particular have taken it upon themselves to defend Christian mores in the face of what they perceive as an increasingly self-absorbed and permissive social order. However, this is not to say that their only concern is the past. Rather, they seek to confront modernity and restructure it to its very core. Finding a ready source of recruits among that segment of the population that has benefited least from the country's economic development, fundamentalists have challenged head-on the "morality" of fornication in general and the practices of sexual minorities in particular.

Still, this is not to suggest that there is only one stream of fundamentalist thought. Most notably, there are significant differences between Fundamentalists and Roman Catholic beliefs. Inter alia, Protestants reject the authority of the Pope, priestly celibacy, the divinity of the Virgin Mary, and the presence of images in church. Whether or not these difference are important in and of themselves—after all, only one of the young people interviewed was able to distinguish between Protestant and Catholic religious doctrine—it is clear that the Protestant churches are closely allied with (and funded by) the American religious right, and as such have adopted many of that movement's views on such subjects as feminism, homosexuality, scientific progress, and family planning. Indeed, one might even go so far as to argue that evangelical Protestants in Costa Rica are *more* doctrinaire and inflexible with respect to sexual matters than their Roman Catholic counterparts.

As one might imagine, fundamentalists place great stress upon the extent to which modern society has abandoned traditional Christian morality. In the words of a study participant who is also the leader of a Christian youth movement, "These days . . . promiscuity is a terrible problem, especially because we live in a world that encourages it. Homosexuality is widespread in today's society." It is obvious that most of the young Protestants whom we interviewed have internalized a highly essentialist understanding of "appropriate" sexual roles and relations. For example, consider the following statements by Alexandra:

- "I believe the natural order of things was established by God. That's why you shouldn't start trying to change things."
- "By imposing His law, God's aim was to eliminate the filth and impurities within us."
- "Temptation can only be avoided by carefully following established norms."
- "God made man and woman so that they would complement each other in marriage."
- "If it's part of God's plan that man and woman be together, there shouldn't anything different."

Similarly, fundamentalists are clearly distrustful of sexual pleasure in all of its forms. To quote Jonathan:

I believe sex is bad; people go berserk doing filthy things. That's why I find sex disgusting and prefer only to give kisses. . . . Young people surrender to pleasure too easily. Sexual urges are very strong in young people; that's where all vice comes from. Sin is everywhere—it's like a current that flows

and drags everything down with it. It's very strong and difficult to stop.

Of course, closely related to the opinions expressed above is the
zeal with which evangelical Christians denounce the principle of
gender equality. Their disdain for the latter was made abundantly
clear during the course of the focus group sessions, where it blended
into manifestations of blatant misogyny and homophobia:

- "Women are characterized by softness and men by strength.
  That's the way it should be and it shouldn't be changed. What
  we need to do is develop the qualities that are innate within
  each sex."
- "As far as femininity and masculinity are concerned, women
  are more delicate; they don't go around lifting weights or
  heavy bags. Men are stronger. That's a basic biological distinction."
- "The wife should be submissive. In a Christian marriage it's
  the man that's boss."
- "When women go around dressed in really tight-fitting mini-
  skirts or T-shirts, I find it offensive. It irritates me."
- "I believe that in societies where women are more liberated
  there are more homosexuals, because men have a harder time
  relating to women in these places."

This last statement is an especially telling one, since the speaker
is attempting to draw a link between female assertiveness on one
hand and male homosexuality on the other. However, while it is
clear that fundamentalists see both as "deviant" to the extent that
they challenge traditional Christian morality, there can be little
doubt that their condemnation of homosexuality is particular severe, as is amply shown by the comments below:

- "By destroying their bodies, these young homosexuals have
  also destroyed their souls."
- "My experience with homosexuals leads me to believe they're
  negative people."
- "They're defensive, secretive fault-finders, they debase themselves; they pretend to be happy but they only sow discord."

- "It's difficult to be with them; they always try to disguise them-selves because they feel bad and it's because they're flawed."

AIDS, from this perspective, is considered a divine punishment imposed upon (and spread by) homosexuals because of their sinful behavior:

- "AIDS is . . . a warning. There is a divine plan, a certain order; if men don't comply with it, they're going to be punished."
- "We knew the AIDS problem was coming; it's written in the Bible. The thing is people don't know it, they ignore it. In a world like ours, so full of evil, destruction, men kill each other, there are vices, homosexuality. That's why AIDS came."
- "The other day there was a special program on television where homosexuals were shown on the street kissing and hug-ging each other, touching each other's buttocks. Many of them have AIDS and live together because they're not afraid of any-thing, not even death or God."

Given their views on the origin of the AIDS epidemic, it is not surprising that many of the young fundamentalists who participated in the study were also opposed to the ethos of scientific enquiry, particularly when the latter calls into question biblical assertions:

- "We have nothing; Jesus has converted us. It's a mystery—it has no rational explanation. Psychologists can't do anything; they can't even reach the Spirit. You can be intellectually and academically accomplished, but if you can't reach the uncon-scious, that is the Spirit, your profession is useless."
- "I think what's really important is God's word . . . science can only help."
- "God alone can cure the Spirit. I have friends who study psychol-ogy and they can reach a certain point, but when they can't do any more, they tell them to go read the Bible."

Of course, messages such as these are appealing to those whose socioeconomic marginalization prevents them from overcoming the problems that they, along with their communities, are facing. This explains why the Pentecostal Church has won over as many followers as it has in Villa del Mar. Quite simply, its uncompromising and activist stance on issues such as drugs, prostitution, adultery, and other "deviant" behaviors is precisely what its adherents expect from their church.

As well, many find the grassroots leadership style of evangelical Christianity appealing, especially when contrasted with the extremely hierarchical and elitist management structure of the Catholic Church. Not only are individuals who have little opportunity to take charge in their day-to-day lives given a chance to become religious leaders in their own right, but many are also attracted by the genuinely spontaneous and participatory nature of church services themselves.

Along similar lines, it should be noted that, despite strongly patriarchal tendencies within most fundamentalist churches, they do offer women somewhat greater scope to play leadership roles than in Roman Catholicism. This, combined with their attacks upon male infidelity and those who shirk their responsibilities as husbands and fathers, helps to explain why Protestant fundamentalism is so popular among female residents of Villa del Mar.

Turning to the question of how successful evangelical Christianity has been in promoting premarital celibacy among young people, there can be little doubt that most members of such churches do indeed plan to abstain from sex until their wedding day. However, the same might be said of devout Roman Catholics, and, as our in-depth interviews made clear, not all fundamentalist youth are successful in avoiding the temptations of sexual activity prior to marriage.

Leidy is typical in this regard. She is nineteen years of age and a longtime member of an Adventist congregation, and her sex education—both at home and at church—has been limited to vague warnings concerning the "dangers" of sex and the importance of "saving" herself for her future husband. The adults in her life have sought to ensure that she does save herself by carefully monitoring her activities. As she put it, "I was never allowed to go to dances, wear makeup, or go out with boys."

Given this information vacuum, Leidy learned about sex elsewhere, from girlfriends at school and from boys on the street. "They were very clever," Leidy admitted, and before long she (and many of her friends as well) had a "secret" boyfriend of whom her mother and church were completely ignorant. However, knowing nothing about contraceptives and safe sex, not only was she soon pregnant, but, once she had revealed her condition to her boyfriend, she was single as well, as he quickly left her to avoid having to support the child once it was born. Although she is the first to admit that she made a mistake, she feels that this is in large part due to the fact that she "had no one to talk to about sex." Needless to say, this has made her somewhat resentful toward her church: "I don't believe women have to remain virgin until marriage. Many young people do it all the time—it's not something you can avoid."

Chapter 7

Assimilation of Gender Discourses

Patriarchy is so firmly entrenched in the West that most people take it for granted. However, this does not alter the fact that it is a gender-based system of domination, whose existence directly benefits men at the same time that it exploits and demeans women.

In the relatively underdeveloped countries of Latin America, patriarchal social relations are more in evidence than they are in Europe or North America, where women have been more successful in countering gender discrimination in their daily lives. Costa Rican women, for example, continue to be treated as second-class citizens, the victims of a culture of "machismo" that denigrates the "feminine" while celebrating all things "masculine."

Needless to say, instilling macho values and norms in children begins at an early age, and consists in the first instance of socializing them into accepting the view that men and women are mirror reflections of one another: one is strong, the other weak; one is aggressive, the other passive, one is rational, the other emotional; one is a breadwinner, the other a homemaker. Of course, once these tenets have been accepted as fact, it is but a short step to the "self-evident" view that men complement women (and vice versa), and thus that heterosexual union is the natural state of being for humankind.

Of course, despite the enthusiasm with which many Costa Rican men embrace machismo, the patriarchal system did not originate in this country. Rather, its roots lie far in the past, obscured by the mists of history and subject to continuing debate among scholars in a wide range of fields. Although it would require a book in itself to do justice to the complex arguments put forth by these writers, one might nonetheless refer to Engels' (1970) *The Origin of the Family, Private Property, and the State*. Although it was first published more than a century ago, its line of reasoning is plausible, and has provided the basis for much subsequent writing on this topic.

Engels argues that prehistoric societies were characterized by systems of governance that were once matriarchal and communist and, despite the existence of a sexual division of labor, women's status was in no way inferior to that of their male counterparts. However, all this changed as agriculture replaced gathering and hunting as the principal means of subsistence, with men taking it upon themselves to keep any surplus generated, and, ultimately, to pass it along to their descendants. As the locus of sexual power shifted, matriarchal governance structures fell increasingly into disuse, to be replaced by ones grounded in patrilineal succession and patriarchal control.

Engels' thesis was greatly developed by feminist scholars in the 1970s and 1980s, who took it upon themselves to engage in further analysis and interpretation of the origins of female subordination and exploitation in Western societies. Many of these writers posited a biological basis for patriarchy. Scherfey (1970), for example, sought to explain the domination of women by men in terms of the woman's capacity to experience multiple orgasms and her capacity to perform with more partners (no need of keeping an erection). Within this frame of reference, women were subordinated in order to circumscribe and control their procreative potential. A similar position was advanced by Susan Brownmiller (1976), who argued that women's oppression derives from their relative physical weakness. In this view, patriarchy's roots can be traced to the moment man first realized that he could use his sexual organ to rape woman.

Others, meanwhile, placed their emphasis somewhat differently, downplaying the importance of biology while highlighting instead the role of a changing political economy. In a particularly notable example, Gerda Lerner (1990) makes the case in *The Creation of Patriarchy* that it was women's subordination at the hands of men that provided the basis for men's subsequent domination of nature and other human societies.

Finally, it should be noted that some feminist scholars have gone so far as to reject the notion that there is any biological basis for patriarchy at all. The work of Monique Witting (1971) is typical of this school of thought. Not only does she contend that all sex roles and relations are socially constructed, but that even supposedly immutable physical processes (such as childbirth and hormone production) are responsive to changing cultural contexts. Thus, analysis of the patriarchal system must be grounded in political rather than anatomical explanations.

This discussion certainly underscores the difficulty of arriving at any clearcut explanation of patriarchy's origins. However, be this as it may, there can be little doubt that it remains a potent force in Costa Rica and elsewhere, subjugating and oppressing women while at the same time dictating the bounds of the "normal" in all matters pertaining to sex roles and relations.

HOW ARE SEX ROLES INTERNALIZED?

From a very early age, boys and girls are taught how to act, think, and speak in ways that are "appropriate" to their gender. Their teachers are many, ranging from parents, siblings, and peers to television, popular music, and magazines. Not only are these messages ubiquitous and multivariate, but they are constantly reinforced through the threat of ridicule, humiliation, and physical violence should an individual fail to abide by them.

The internalization process is both conscious and unconscious, starting at home and continuing throughout the life course. Yadira Calvo (in Berrón, 1995), a distinguished Costa Rican feminist, recalls learning her subordinate role as a child, in the small details of daily life: in the amount of food served to men and women (the latter are served less), or in processes of household decision making (all the important decisions are made by men). Calvo's experiences are validated by the findings of academic studies of the impact of gender upon adults' perception of babies and young children. That is to say, there is a strong tendency to see girls as passive and boys as aggressive, regardless of the actual behavior of the children in question (Kaschak, 1993).

Other key sites involved in the process of gender internalization include school and church. In schools, this is demonstrated in the way that teachers devote more attention to the boys under their care than the girls. At the same time, girls tend to be interrupted more often when they are speaking, and are given fewer chances to comment or ask questions. As for church, women's subordination is rendered self-evident by the fact that they are banned from entering the priesthood, along with frequent exhortations from the pulpit that they fulfill their God-given role as wives and mothers.

Taken together, these messages serve not only to ensure that individuals comply with the dominant gender order, but they are implicated as well in the creation of a psychology of gender, whereby men and women position themselves according to a particular set of engendered identities. Needless to say, once they are internalized in this way, they become very difficult to change.

PUBLIC AWARENESS OF GENDER
AND THE IMPULSE FOR CHANGE

Patriarchal gender relations have been a fixture of Costa Rican society since the earliest days of Spanish rule, and have long provoked resistance on the part of the country's women. While some have denounced incidents of rape and incest committed against them, and publicly demanded compensation (Molina Jiménez and Palmer, 1994), others' resistance has been more private in orientation, embodying self-empowerment or a refusal to become complicit in the reproduction of the existing gender order.

However, despite the undoubted importance of these women's actions, knowledge about them has been lost or suppressed as a result of mainstream scholars' obsession with *his*tory, in which marginal or discordant voices are cast aside as irrelevant. Thus, at the moment that feminist writers purposely set out to reclaim the past through the lens of *her*story, the question of whether women ever resisted patriarchy was replaced by the question of when it became a matter of public concern.

In Costa Rica, one might argue that the first public manifestation of women's power occurred in 1923, as the country's nascent Feminist League embarked upon a campaign to secure women's right to vote. Despite the League's eventual success—female enfranchisement became a reality following the 1948 civil war—it was never able to broaden its base of support beyond a relatively small community of urban intellectuals. Thus, it was not until the 1970s, with the wide-scale incorporation of women into the wage labor force and the rebirth of a national feminist movement energized by the gains made by women in North America and Europe, that feminist ideas began to take root among a broader cross-section of Costa Rica's female population (Berrón, 1995).

Not only was it at this time that reference began to be made to the country's "gender problem," but there was also growing recognition of the fact that gender identities, far from being immutable and static, are negotiable and subject to change. Needless to say, this marked a significant departure from the past, and as such its origins warrant further discussion.

Few developments were more important in this regard than the government's decision in the 1970s to make contraceptives widely available to Costa Rica's female population. There was a growing concern that large families of ten or more children were no longer appropriate in a country that was attempting to abandon its agricultural past in favor of an industrialized, urbanized future. Thus, in an attempt to reduce family size, clinics and hospitals across the country opened their doors to thousands of women, offering them a range of birth control options, including most notably the Pill.

Whether or not this intervention had its desired effect, there can be little doubt that it had a significant impact upon the women themselves. Not only were they brought together in clinic waiting rooms where they could discuss issues and problems they faced in common, empowering themselves in the process, but their newfound control over the number of babies they bore gave them a degree of autonomy in their relationships with men that would have been unimaginable to their mothers and grandmothers. For the first time in Costa Rican history, women had a tool to redefine motherhood and gender expectations and were doing so with others in the context of the consciousness-raising process taking place in the clinic waiting rooms.

Without wishing to exaggerate the impact of contraceptive availability upon the patriarchal system itself, one might nonetheless argue that it served to call into question certain fundamental assumptions regarding women's "proper" role in life. Was it merely to produce children and provide sexual and personal services to a working husband? Increasingly, there were those who argued that it was not, with university-based feminists taking the lead in attacking the sexist stereotyping that was endemic in almost all areas of Costa Rican society.

At the same time that these activists were engaged in campaigns against beauty contests, female poverty, and male violence, ordinary women across the country were beginning to make changes in their own lives, whether going out to find work in the paid workforce, or demanding that their men do more to help them with domestic chores. However, despite their success in undermining some of the assumptions and generalizations that had served them so ill in the past, those assumptions were rapidly replaced by new ones that were no less harmful to the cause of sexual equality.

For example, discourses that portrayed women as nothing more than baby-making machines gave way to ones which emphasized the complexities of motherhood, and women's key responsibility for the psychological and moral development of their children. Along similar lines, the view that a wife is nothing more than her husband's servant was abandoned in favor of one which cast women in the role of passionate lover and understanding companion, with all of the duties and burdens that this position imposes.

Still, regardless of these developments, it is clear that men have been put on the defensive by women's growing assertiveness and independence. Although this has led to some concessions on their part—for example, in their willingness to take on certain household responsibilities—they have also become more demanding of their spouses in the area of emotional support, and ready to blame them for their children's problems. It should also be noted that most Costa Rican women have refrained from pressing for radical change in dominant sex roles and relations. Thus, even though there is widespread agreement that patriarchy remains a force to be reckoned with, few would go so far as to advocate the dismantling of the institutions of marriage and motherhood in their entirety. In this way, one might argue that the country's feminists are firmly grounded in the liberal camp, and that there is little support for a radical feminist program of revolutionary change in the way that women and men relate to one another.

MALE GENDER DISCOURSES

The dominant gender order among young Costa Ricans has undergone significant changes over the course of recent years. Thus, although young men are aware of the unambiguously patriarchal nature of their parents and grandparents' relationships, they have sought to follow a somewhat different path.

Drawing upon findings from the in-depth interviews, male adolescents' assimilation of gender principles has produced an orientation that might best be described as one of "enlightened despotism." That is, despite arguing that men possess attributes which women lack, and thus that male superiority can be taken for granted, respondents also sought to emphasize the importance of using power responsibly. In this sense, their view is reminiscent of the reform-minded citizens of ancient Greece who advocated the use of "temperance" in men's dealings with women, thereby marking a departure from the highly dictatorial relationship that had been the norm in the past.

Although the reasons for this evolution in young men's attitudes are clearly multidimensional, one might nonetheless point to two factors that appear to be especially important in this regard. On one hand, women's struggle for equality, combined with increased rates of participation in the paid workforce, have clearly had an impact on men's assimilation of feminist principles. On the other, men's heightened sensitivity to the dangers posed by HIV/AIDS and other STDs have prompted many to look askance at machismo's emphasis upon proving one's virility through sex with multiple partners.

However, this is not to say that Costa Rican men have internalized a discourse of full equality between the sexes. Instead, as already discussed, the dominant discourse has merely shifted its emphasis, with certain restrictions being lifted (e.g., on women holding certain jobs) while new demands are imposed. Foremost among the latter is the expectation that a wife, besides caring for her husband's children, will also act as his therapist, being "understanding" and "supportive" while helping him resolve his emotional crises. This role has been extended to encompass offspring as well. No longer is it deemed acceptable for mothers to attend merely to their children's physical needs; safeguarding the latter's psychological development is now seen as being equally important, with responsibility for any lapses in a child's behavior placed squarely on the shoulders of his or her mother.

Despite the assumption that women can fulfill all that is expected of them while receiving little or no emotional support in return, most of the young men who participated in the study believed women to be the naturally weaker sex, both physically and psychologically. This is demonstrated in Juan's comment that women should not go out alone "because they might be assaulted," or in Jonathan's recollection of being beaten as a child, and being told that he "should take the pain like a man."

This tendency to associate weakness with women has led male participants to reject any behavior that might be considered "feminine." For example, Carlos indicated that cooking was unmanly because "it's a woman's job." Meanwhile, Jonathan reported being told by his mother that men are meant to "go out and earn a living," and thus should not be required to perform domestic tasks. Maikol distinguishes men and women on the basis of whether or not it is appropriate for them to cry. Finally, Jorge and Donaldo differentiate the sexes according to personal habits and appearance, with the latter arguing that only women should have long hair, while the former stated that he found it odd when men devoted time to "womanly things," such as dressing fashionably or grooming themselves.

Still, it is clear that young men's definition of what constitutes "womanly things" is undergoing something of a transformation. In particular, there appears to be growing acceptance, at least among some of the interview participants, of male involvement in activities related to the social reproduction of the household, such as cooking and cleaning. Thus, despite the fact that his father does not help with domestic chores, Kenneth indicated that he regularly sweeps and washes the floor. Along similar lines, Guillermo stated that doing housework does not "bother" or "embarrass" him.

Sports and the workplace are two additional areas where there is evidence of a more progressive attitude on the part of some of the male participants. Mainor, for one, suggested that women should be able to "study and work in whatever field they like. These days there are women bus drivers and women mechanics." Others agreed, with Guillermo and Aaron stating that even construction work should not be off-limits to those women who wish to pursue it. Questions about sports elicited a similar response. Respondents felt it was unfair to prevent women from participating in certain sports solely on the basis of their sex, with the only exception being boxing, because (according to Aaron) "there's this idea about women being too feminine for this sort of thing."

As one might imagine, this point is important, underlining as it does the fact that there are still some forms of behavior that the young men interviewed will not tolerate among their female friends and lovers.

Foul language is the first such area all the more so if the words in question are related to sex or sexual organs. For example, as David made clear, a "decent" woman would never dare say such things as "let's fuck" or "let me suck your dick." Most other participants agreed, with Santiago going so far as to say that he broke up with his girlfriend because "she let dirty words slip out."

Sexually forward or aggressive women were similarly reviled by male research participants. On one hand, there is a dim view of women who ask men out, with Aaron in particular arguing that women should never take the initiative and should always be more "conservative." On the other, there was widespread hostility toward women who had extramarital affairs or multiple partners. Although some tempered their criticism by acknowledging that they expected women to adhere to a higher standard of behavior, there was a clear consensus among the participants that failure to meet this standard could not be tolerated. Thus, Danny argued that women who initiate sex risk being raped, while David referred to such individuals as "holes" and "pigs." Finally, Donaldo stated that women should resist the urge to engage in intercourse because they might get pregnant and have to support the child.

However, as long as women observe these interdictions, it was generally felt that men should exercise their power magnanimously, and treat members of the "weaker" sex with respect and consideration. Luis, for example, stressed that women should not be treated as "objects" or "slaves," and that it was men's duty to "protect" their female friends and relatives from potential aggressors. In similar fashion, Mainor suggested that men should choose their words carefully and not be "coarse" when in female company, a point echoed by Carlos, who emphasized the importance of always being respectful, courteous, and affectionate toward women.

Although there was general consensus among male participants that they must act responsibly toward the women in their lives, most went on to say that they were generally happy with dominant sex roles and relations. Thus, even though Frederico was cognizant of men's "authoritarian" tendencies, he indicated that he was "quite satisfied" with his upbringing and the way in which he related to women. Aaron, despite claiming that he was not a partisan of machismo himself, felt that it would be unwise to attempt to alter existing sex roles, since this would be viewed "unfavorably" by many segments of society. Conversely, both Guillermo and Jorge, even as they argued that much of men and women's behavior is ingrained and thus difficult to change, said that they wished men could give freer rein to their emotions.

Of course, whether or not young men have any interest in moving away from macho forms of sexual expression, in many cases they are being forced to do so by the prospect of contracting HIV/ AIDS. For the majority of interview participants—even those who were eighteen or nineteen years of age—the dangers posed by this disease were such that they abstained from sex altogether, even if this meant being unable to boast about their virility to their friends. Thus, while Aaron explained his virginity by noting that "abstinence helps to avoid risks," Jorge went so far as to claim that he never even masturbates, so great is his fear of HIV infection and God's wrath.

FEMALE GENDER DISCOURSES

In examining women's understanding of these issues, a somewhat different picture emerges. Although female participants were in broad agreement with their male counterparts on the biological roots of gender, and in particular the notion that men and women's roles in life are opposite yet complementary, in no way did they believe that this justified women's subordination.

Thus, even as they acknowledged men's superior strength, courage, and stamina, the young women interviewed went on to argue in favor of a gender order based on specialization rather than domination, in which men and women devote themselves to different tasks and responsibilities and, in so doing, enhance the quality of one another's lives.

What does gender "specialization" entail? As one might imagine, it is firmly grounded within the dominant paradigm, with several participants arguing that hormonal differences between the sexes, together with women's central role in biological reproduction, dictate what the latter should and should not do. As Susana put it, "Women are more maternal. . . . They have to stay in the house because they're the ones who get pregnant and have to care for the children. That's natural and cannot be changed." Other female participants agreed, with Adriana arguing that "since women conceive, they're made for housework," while Diana suggested that fondness for children is "in women's genes, it's totally natural."

However, if the young women who participated in the study were united in stressing the key importance of maternal "instinct" in women's lives, there was far less agreement on the implications of that instinct. Thus, while some adopted an extreme position and stated that women should devote themselves exclusively to domestic activities, others were more open-minded, arguing that there should be few or no restrictions on women's career choices, with the possible exception of policing and construction work. Needless to say, those who were more conservative in their outlook tended to be equally uncomfortable with women's involvement in sports. Wendoly was particularly adamant in this regard, stressing that soccer, baseball, and basketball were all activities that should be off-limits to women.

Still, despite the traditionalism of some of the research participants, all felt that men should play an active part in child care and daily household chores. Hilda, for one, believes that husbands owe it to their wives to take responsibility for half of this work: "I think that if a woman can do the household chores, so can a man." In similar fashion, both Adriana and Tatiana emphasized that housework should be shared equally among men and women, with Adriana going so far as to argue that men should help cook as well.

An egalitarian outlook was also in evidence when discussing questions of mobility. That is, female participants strongly disagreed with the view, espoused by many of their male counterparts, that restrictions should be placed upon women's freedom of movement. Thus, Tatiana said that she gets irritated when her mother asks her father for permission to leave their home, when she knows full well that her father needs no such permission himself. In a similar vein, Hilda expressed dismay at her mother's submissiveness, and the fact that she is "stuck inside the house when [her father] goes out whenever he likes." Finally, Maria indicated that she does not understand why she has less freedom than the male members of her family. As she put it, "They do whatever they please and if they want they don't even have to come home to sleep, yet I have to ask permission for everything."

Of course, closely related to the issue of mobility rights is that of female objectification. As one might imagine, there was widespread revulsion toward men who partake of pornography, sexual violence, or other activities that debase women. Wendoly, for example, indicated that she feels disgust whenever a "man makes insinuations by gripping his crotch." In parallel fashion, Daisy has little respect for her male classmates who continuously boast about their sexual exploits, and is sickened by the way in which they treat the sex act as though it were "like drinking a glass of water."

Needless to say, sexual violence aroused a similar degree of revulsion, with several participants indicating that they would never tolerate it in the context of a relationship. Wendoly went furthest in this regard, relating the story of how she had been raped by her father's friend, a violation that left her with feelings of great "resentment" and a "thorn in the heart."

However, in spite of the views expressed above, it is clear that the young women interviewed do support key aspects of the patriarchal gender system, if only for fear of what would take its place. In the words of Dunia, "I don't know what would happen if there were no differences between men and women and we were all alike; I'd worry that we would no longer have any rapport with each other."

Thus, the majority of female participants had little wish to change the way in which men and women interacted on a day-to-day basis. Wendoly, for one, felt it was very important that men be masculine and women feminine: "It's horrible to see a woman who's aggressive and not submissive" or, for that matter, a man who dresses up "like a woman." Daisy shares this view, arguing that "there should be differences" between the sexes, and that it behooves women to "show off their femininity and dress in tight clothing." Others agreed, all the while stressing the unsightliness of men who choose to dress in an "unmasculine" fashion. In Susana's estimation such men are usually "faggots," just as women who pay little attention to their personal appearance are probably "dykes."

Sex and courtship initiation are two additional areas in which female participants were happy with the existing distribution of roles and responsibilities. With regard to courtship in particular, there was a general consensus that women should always wait for the man to take the initiative. Otherwise, as Daisy put it, they would be considered "very fresh" at best, and prostitutes at worst, since "only hookers ask men out." Along similar lines, the majority of young women also felt that men should be the ones to play a leading role in the sex act itself, since they were thought to be more knowledgeable in these matters than their female counterparts. Tatiana, for example, felt it was important for men to "help" their wives on the night of their wedding, as "the woman is usually very nervous." Leidy agreed with this perspective, arguing that men will inevitably have more experience "because nobody could care less whether he's a virgin or not on his wedding night."

Given these statements, is one to conclude that young women are generally happy with the manner in which the men in their lives interact with them? Although there is clearly some appreciation for men's forwardness in the realm of relationships, the bulk of participants went on to say that they wished their men were more communicative and expressive. Hilda, for one, said that although she is attracted to strong, masculine men, she would "like them to be more affectionate and giving." Likewise, several participants commented upon the tendency among men to treat their girlfriends as inanimate objects, with scant regard for the latter's feelings. Thus, as Leidy made clear, there is a need for men to counter this state of affairs by "surrendering" to their emotions and being more giving in the context of their relationships.

Indeed, in many respects Leidy's perspective is typical of female participants' view of gender relations in general. That is, even as they are willing to accept certain premises set forth within the existing gender system, for example in the areas of dress and interpersonal relations, they would like to mitigate or erase those aspects which they find most harmful, such as sexual violence and objectification. Obviously, this is a liberal position rather than a radical one, yet it is seen by the young women who took part in the study as the strategy that is most likely to produce results without running the risk of shattering their families and relationships.

GENDER DISCOURSES IN THE COMMUNITIES

Considerable effort has already been devoted to the task of comparing and contrasting the cultural contexts within which young people live out their lives in the two communities under study. However, one issue that has not been discussed thus far is that of the relationship between *cacheros* and *playos,* two figures who are well-known to Villa del Mar youth, yet have no equivalent in Villa del Sol.

Who are they? Quite simply, a *cachero* is a masculine, seemingly heterosexual man who engages in active anal intercourse with other men, usually *playos.* These latter individuals are, as Alberto put it, men who "dress like women and wish they were one." David is typical in this regard: he enjoys passive anal sex and dressing in drag, and would eventually like to become a transvestite.

What is important to bear in mind, however, is that Villa del Mar residents do not consider *cacheros* to be homosexual. Even David, whose partners include both married and single men, stressed this point: "The guys I sleep with are real men." Other young people agree, with Kenneth describing a recent trip to the beach when he and his friends came across two men having sex. However, rather than referring to the parties involved as gay, Kenneth characterized them instead as a "man fucking a *playo.*"

As one might imagine, there is no such distinction in Villa del Sol, where *playos* are simply men who sleep with other men; whether one is the active or the passive partner is considered immaterial. Of course, such a view is grounded in a rational-scientific understanding of sexual orientation, in which homosexuality is only a deviation from the heterosexual norm. As we emphasize in the pages that follow, this translates into significantly different gender discourses in the two communities. Whereas in Villa del Sol emphasis is placed upon gender "psychology" when attempting to make sense of men and women's relationships, in Villa del Mar attention is focused instead upon the "activity" or "passivity" of particular individuals.

Gender Discourses in Villa del Mar

Economic stagnation and chronic unemployment are defining characteristics of Villa del Mar. In this environment, men are faced with the prospect of joblessness for much of the year, while women are forced to find wage-paying work themselves to make ends meet, either in the service sector, or in local *maquiladoras** and tuna-processing plants.

Needless to say, economic marginalization has had far-reaching effects upon the community's social fiber, as attested by high levels of family violence, divorce, and single parenthood among its population. Indeed, so poor are the prospects of many of the town's male inhabitants and so great is their level of alienation and anger that women will often prefer to leave their partners (either for another man or to live by themselves with their children) rather than stay in an abusive relationship.

However, the degree of economic independence many women in Villa del Mar enjoy has not translated into heightened respect for the rights of women in general. Rather, one might argue that the reverse is true, given that the community is characterized by a more "traditional" gender order than Villa del Sol, where feminism has made considerable headway, particularly among the community's younger members.

What, then, of gender relations in the town? Villa del Mar's residents subscribe to an ideology centered upon the body and its physical activities. Within this model, women and men are defined according to their relative aggressivity or passivity, with roles and activities appropriate to each. In women's case, they are required to act as caregivers and nurturers, providing a range of personal services to their children and husbands. In men's case, they are expected to be the family's breadwinner and leader, and to protect it from external threats and dangers. Underpinning this division of labor are well-defined rules and conventions outlining the bounds of "appropriate" behavior. Thus, women do not need to be told that they should act, dress, and talk in a "feminine" fashion, just as men do not have to be reminded of the importance of always behaving in a suitably "masculine" manner.

It is precisely in this context that the *cachero* derives his significance. That is, Villa del Mar encompasses a worldview in which

---

*Export-oriented factories where workers only assemble parts rather than make them.

sexuality, rather than being defined through the elaboration of a series of psychological attributes (as is the case in Villa del Sol), is grounded instead in the dichotomization of dominator and dominated. Within this frame of reference, all those who are aggressive and dominate others are necessarily men, while those who are passive and dominated are by definition women.

Given this perspective, the object of desire, be it man or woman, becomes less important than the identity of the subject: *playos,* because of their femininity, are understood to be women in men's bodies, just as "butch" lesbians are thought to be men in women's bodies. Meanwhile, those who behave in a manner "appropriate" to their gender—such as *cacheros* and feminine lesbians—are labeled heterosexual, regardless of whom their lovers happen to be.

Of course, it is no coincidence that this model is the predominant one in Villa del Mar. Since it is a community in crisis, whose menfolk feel emasculated and threatened because they cannot provide for their families, the men compensate for their own sense of powerlessness by dominating others physically. That is, men are encouraged to prove themselves by using violence to subjugate those around them, most notably their wives and children. Inordinately high levels of physical aggression were apparent throughout the research process, with young people relating any number of stories of beatings, sexual and physical abuse, rape, and incest.

To illustrate the degree to which violence has become part of young men's everyday lives, it is useful to consider the following statement by Kenneth, who was explaining when one can legitimately force oneself upon a woman: "Sometimes the eyes tell you. They say no, but their eyes and their body language say yes. In cases like that, it's okay to use force."

Gender Discourses in Villa del Sol

Not only is Villa del Sol a more affluent community than Villa del Mar, but it embodies a gender order that is itself conditioned by economic mobility, high levels of educational attainment, and a male population whose ready access to employment opportunities facilitates the fulfillment of breadwinning obligations to their families.

While these characteristics have undoubtedly played a role in discouraging divorce and separation in the town, they have also contributed to the elaboration of an understanding of "appropriate" gender roles and relations which stands in sharp contrast to that which is predominant in Villa del Mar.

How so? Whereas gender discourses in Villa del Mar focus on physical strength and the active-passive dichotomy, in Villa del Sol emphasis is placed instead upon the interplay of opposing (yet complementary) "psychologies." From this perspective, women are women not so much because of their supposed "passivity," but rather on account of their distinctly "feminine" mentality and thought processes. It is precisely because of men and women's different mentalities that the latter are thought best-suited for care-giving and nurturing tasks, and the former for activities that are competitive, arduous, or intellectually challenging.

The complementarity of this gender system should be obvious. It assumes that the mental development of men and women, whether by virtue of education, hormones, or peer expectations, produces incomplete minds that need each other if they are to become whole. However, despite its tendency to damn as "deviant" those who do not fall neatly into one category or the other, the model is nonetheless flexible in the face of changing realities. The reason is simple: male and female roles are interrelated. Thus, to the extent that being male in Villa del Sol means simply not being female, women can take on new roles or redefine existing ones without necessarily undermining the premises upon which the gender model is based.

Indeed, gains have been made in this area. No longer are household chores the sole purview of wives and daughters, as men are showing themselves increasingly willing (even if reluctantly) to assist in meal preparation and child care. Similarly, women can now pursue their studies or become career-minded professionals without risking the wrath of their partners. Still, this is not to say that gender discourses have ceased to be oppressive. For example, even though it is no longer unthinkable for young women in Villa del Sol to engage in premarital sex, they are still forced to contend with a pernicious double standard. As Hilda put it:

> If a man goes around with a lot of chicks it doesn't matter, but a woman must make herself be respected. However, society is opening up and a woman who takes the initiative is no longer

considered a slut. Still, men have to "fuck" a lot of chicks in order to be considered manly.

Women are also aware that they are the ones who will pay the price should they be unlucky enough to become pregnant within the context of a premarital relationship. At best, their family will forgive their "mistake" and continue to lend support; at worst, they will be abandoned by their boyfriends and left to fend for themselves. Indeed, there are some who might argue that, at the same time that middle-class women are gaining access to new rights and new possibilities, their partners are placing new burdens upon them (e.g., in the area of emotional support), undermining the gains made in the process. Thus, for a woman like Maria, true gender equality remains a faraway and elusive goal: "What I am saying is that women suffer more than men, it's always the woman who gives more love, and then we are ridiculed for it. It would have been better to have been born a man and not suffer so much."

Chapter 8

Assimilation of Scientific Discourses

Given the complexity inherent within the sexual discourses of science, arising as they do from any number of disciplinary contexts, it would scarcely be feasible for us to attempt to make sense of all of them in this chapter. Rather, we will focus instead upon that which is most relevant to the work at hand, namely the discourses that fall under the rubric of "reproductive health."

As one might imagine, this discourse is heavily influenced by the biomedical model, in which "problems," be they an overabundance of teenage pregnancies or the spread of STDs, can be corrected through the application of the appropriate "cure." Prescribed by physicians, nurses, or social workers, these cures generally take the form of education and prevention campaigns, in which "scientific" information is mobilized in the fight against diseases (or, in the case of pregnancy, "irresponsible" behavior) and the conditions that facilitate their propagation.

However, before we set out to explore the impact of reproductive health discourses upon Costa Rica's young people, we must first provide some background information. As discussed in Chapter 2, the country's indigenous population is estimated to have been between 20,000 and 30,000 at the time of first contact with the Spanish colonizers. However, disease brought from Europe would soon take its toll, and by 1611 this figure is believed to have dropped to 15,000. It would take close to a century before it returned to its precontact level (Thiel, 1977). In more recent times, of course, the rate of growth accelerated considerably, with the population climbing from 300,000 to 800,000 in the fifty years between 1900 and 1950, and to well over 3 million in the early 1990s (CELADE, 1988).

However one wishes to account for this surge in Costa Rica's population, especially in the post-World War II era, there can be little doubt that state-led industrialization and "modernization" were key contributing factors. In short, this was a period when vaccination campaigns, combined with improved living conditions and access to primary medical care, conspired to slash the country's mortality rate in a dramatic fashion, from 25 per 1,000 in the 1940s to less than 10 per 1,000 in the 1960s (ADC, 1986).

Although much of the ensuing growth was initially absorbed by the countryside, it was not long before the region's carrying capacity was reached, prompting ever-larger numbers of people to relocate from their rural homes to urban areas. To the extent that the nascent industrial sector was unable to provide jobs for the new arrivals, overpopulation became a growing concern for state officials, whose response included the creation of the National Programme for Family Planning and Sex Education in 1968 (since renamed the Reproductive Health Programme).

Consequently, it was at this moment that family planning moved from the private realm to the public, and became a legitimate object for state intervention. With support provided by a number of agencies, including the Ministry of Health, the Costa Rican Social Security Fund, and various nongovernmental organizations, the program gave women access to a range of contraceptive options, as well as providing them with information on the benefits of birth spacing and means of avoiding unwanted pregnancies. Without wishing to downplay the degree of opposition to the program's objectives, it was clearly successful in promoting widespread contraceptive use, as is attested by the fact that Costa Rican women are now more likely to be users of contraceptives than their counterparts anywhere else in Latin America (CCSS, 1994).

However, if state agents achieved their declared aim of reining in an unsustainably high birth rate, their interventions also served to achieve another end, perhaps less welcome, namely that of exposing Costa Rican society to a plethora of new discourses related to sex, sexuality, and reproductive health. Not only were technical advances in these areas widely discussed in the mainstream media, but the country became immersed in a series of debates over the morality of such practices as contraceptive use, abortion, and sterilization. As one might imagine, religious groups took the lead in denouncing any hint of liberalization in these areas, and there can be little doubt that their opposition explains, at least in part, the continuing illegality of abortion and sterilization in all cases except those in which the patient's own health is at risk.

Once matters of sex and sexuality had entered the public sphere, the terms of debate soon broadened to encompass other contentious issues as well, adolescent sexual practices most notable among them. This was the time when experts "discovered" the dangers inherent in young people's sexual impulses, with the case of teenage pregnancy cited as a key example. That is, not only was there thought to be a physical risk to mother and child, but their emotional and psychological well-being were considered to be in great danger as well.

Of course, this is part of a larger movement, reflective of broad socioeconomic changes taking place in the country as a whole, away from the notion of "youth" and toward that of "adolescence." Although there had previously been little differentiation between adulthood and youthfulness—after all, this was the time when most people got married, had children (in the case of women), or became apprenticed to a trade (in the case of men)—adolescence was increasingly portrayed as the stage in one's life when one *prepared* oneself for the burdens of adulthood. Thus, it was understood above all to be a waiting period, meant to instill in young people a greater preoccupation with their future as wage earners, consumers, and parents. Needless to say, "waiting" in this context also referred to sexual initiation, with the country's opinion leaders adopting the position that, if individuals were not yet ready to set out on a career and life of their own, how could they be trusted to engage in "responsible" sex?

Still, despite the proliferation of messages regarding the importance of a (relatively) carefree adolescence to individuals' personal development, it is clear that not all young people are able to enjoy this stage in their lives to an equal degree. Poorer families, with fewer resources, simply do not have the luxury of keeping children at home who do not contribute substantively to the social reproduction of the household, just as they cannot afford to send them to university or provide them with the means of embarking upon a profitable career trajectory.

Be this as it may, there can be little doubt that all Costa Rican youth were touched, to a greater or lesser degree, by this new understanding of adolescent sexuality. Beginning in the 1960s, state agents, in association with nongovernmental organizations, launched a series of health programs in the country's secondary schools, at the same time that dominant discourses became increasingly strident in their condemnation of youthful sexual activity. As part of this process, parents were expected to control and monitor their children's activities, while implanting in them the capacity to exercise self-control over their impulses and urges.

Although one might argue that school-based sex education was meant to provide further reinforcement to these messages, the Ministry of Education's efforts in this regard were effectively undermined by vocal criticism on the part of Church authorities, who were strongly opposed to any move that weakened their grip on the moral instruction of the young. As one might imagine, the ensuing debate was both raucous and emotional, as well as progressively broad-based. Should family planning methods be discussed with boys, girls, or both sexes? What about sexual intercourse? Abortion? Homosexuality? Masturbation? What forms of contraceptives are legitimate? Should birth spacing be recommended or not?

Obviously, there are no simple answers to these questions, yet even as religious discourse structured and circumscribed the terms of debate, other, competing discourses were entering the fray. One of these was of course science, which proposed its own wholly secular perspective on sex and sexuality. Another was the street, which offered young people the chance to learn about sex in an environment that was far removed from the disapproving gaze of authority figures.

However, in the 1980s, a new ingredient was introduced into the debate: HIV/AIDS. Not only did its spread to Costa Rica arouse widespread fear and consternation among the population at large, but it also forced state agents, among others, to come to terms with the fact that many adolescents were sexually active, and hence at risk of contracting the virus. Its arrival also had another significant effect, namely that of mobilizing the gay community against homophobic claims that the disease amounted to divine punishment for perverse behavior, in the process making it very difficult to deny the existence of homosexuality in the country, or to pretend that Costa Rica was a model for all its neighbors in the field of human rights.

This last point is especially significant when considered along-side the fact that the government's initial response to HIV/AIDS in 1985 included measures that actively discriminated against sexual minorities, as though infection were the product of identity rather than practice (Madrigal and Schifter, 1990). However, under pres-sure from donor countries and international organizations, state agencies were cajoled into removing overtly homophobic elements from their AIDS programs. While this is not to suggest that these programs ceased to be guided by a conservative ideology—amply attested by the emphasis placed upon abstinence and monogamy as the prevention strategies of choice—the government began to rec-ognize the value in a harm reduction approach. Motivated by fears of an epidemic of disastrous proportions, state agencies began to distribute information on the proper use of condoms, along with other ways that individuals at high risk of infection might protect themselves.

Indeed, it is precisely in this context that HIV/AIDS created the conditions necessary for frank discussion of a host of sex-related subjects that had previously been out-of-bounds as far as polite society and the mainstream media were concerned. Thus, in spite of the alarmist tone adopted by some, there can be little doubt that the public in general was exposed to positions and perspectives (for example, in the area of sexual orientation) that, ten years previously, would never have been allowed to see the light of day. Similarly, once state managers had decided to take an active role in AIDS prevention and education, it became increasingly difficult for them to sanction the dissemination of certain messages (e.g., always practice safe sex) while arbitrarily silencing others (e.g., women have the same right to sexual fulfillment as men).

However, given the extent to which the Church remains a potent political force in Costa Rica, the government has been loath to risk alienating it altogether. Instead, one might argue that the two have reached an unofficial understanding, whereby "illegitimate" prac-tices are tolerated so long as they are not publicized. Female steril-ization is a case in point. Denounced by the Church hierarchy as sinful and unacceptable, it is the contraceptive of choice for Costa

Rican couples (Madrigal, 1994), and is widely available to women in hospitals throughout the country.

SCIENTIFIC DISCOURSES AND YOUNG PEOPLE

Regardless of the state's motives in promoting a "scientific" understanding of sex and sexuality, it is clear that young people have assimilated the latter in the same way that they internalize any other discourse: accept that which is expedient and reject the rest. Indeed, there is little reason to believe that the young people who took part in this study are even aware of the basic tenets of scientific thought. If they were, one presumes that they would be willing to modify their perspective in the face of countervailing evidence. As it stands, however, their support for scientific postulates is limited to those instances where these validate already-held positions and beliefs.

For example, in some of the focus groups, we called into question young people's view of the origins of homosexuality by informing them that there is no scientific basis for the belief that most gay or lesbian individuals are born into dysfunctional families. Although Villa del Mar youth, who generally subscribe to an essentialist understanding of homosexuality in any case, were entirely willing to accept the veracity of this claim, those from Villa del Sol rejected it out of hand, since it was inconsistent with their belief that being gay is the result of environmental factors.

This in turn supports the view that young people's assimilation of scientific discourses is fractured along lines of class and gender, which act similarly to "barriers" or "filters." How they do so and the effects they produce are among the issues which will be addressed in detail in the sections that follow.

Male Discourses in Villa del Sol

As has been suggested in previous chapters, young men in Villa del Sol were among the most likely of all research participants to espouse rational-scientific discourses, and the least likely to have internalized religious ones. Of course, in this connection it is useful to recall that Villa del Sol is a relatively wealthy community, and hence its members have access to monetary, educational, and psychological resources that are quite simply unavailable to their counterparts in Villa del Mar.

Needless to say, these resources, together with the social and educational mobility with which they are associated, have served Villa del Sol's young men well, giving them self-confidence in their reasoning skills and shielding them from the physical dangers that are all too prevalent on the streets in Villa del Mar. While this in turn has made them that much more likely to listen to and act upon "scientific" advice in the area of AIDS or STD prevention, it has also prompted them to emphasize rational thought at the expense of emotions and intuition.

This perspective is evident in their view of the differences between men and women. Making liberal use of Freudian categories and explanations, male participants from Villa del Sol see the sexes as the product of contrasting processes of psychological development, which serve to create adult men and women whose minds are at once opposing yet complementary. Given this view, it does not matter that women are now engaging in activities that were once seen as exclusively male (e.g., attending university), since their femininity is understood to rest elsewhere, for example, in their way of thinking and interacting with others.

Of course, it bears emphasis that young men do not necessarily subscribe to this "scientific" explanation of gender differences because it has been judged to be the most logical or reasonable. Rather, they do so, at least in part, because it offers them a stable worldview and justification for the status quo.

Male participants' self-interest is also discernible in their defense of government-sponsored family planning programs, which they justify through reference to a range of economic arguments. In short, not only did they suggest that large families amounted to a serious financial drain on household resources, but they alluded to the dangers of excessively rapid population growth as well. For example, consider the following statements made by Carlos and Alexandro, respectively:

> Before having a child, you have to plan, you have to know how much money you're going to spend, how many children

you're going to have, and when you have them, what you're going to do.

You have to wait two years to have another child, you have to use contraceptive methods like condoms, the pill and all that shit. Doctors must have some reason for telling us to use them.

Young men also supported safe sexual practices, invoking social and individual responsibility as reasons why one should always use a condom when having sex. As Aaron put it:

Once my sister brought a brochure explaining about condoms and I think that if I hadn't read it I wouldn't know how to use it. I liked it a lot and it helped me learn how to use it. It's a way of planning and preventing health problems, diseases, and pregnancies.

Indeed, despite the fact that not all participants had actually worn a condom, the vast majority were in favor of their use, with individuals offering numerous reasons for their stance, ranging from "the idea appeals to me" to "I must protect myself." Also noteworthy in this regard is the fact that many of the young men suggested that *both* partners should take responsibility for STD prevention, and that it is not simply up to the woman to convince her reluctant mate to wear a condom in spite of himself.

However, by the same token it is clear that cultural barriers to widespread condom use continue to exist in Villa del Sol. That is to say, even though they appear to be readily available in local stores and pharmacies, the majority of participants indicated that they would be too embarrassed to buy them in their community.

Turning to questions related to the spread of HIV/AIDS, our interview and focus group sessions provided ample evidence in support of the view that prevention messages disseminated through the mass media are having an impact upon Costa Rican youth. Thus, young men in Villa del Sol showed themselves to be quite knowledgeable regarding modes of transmission and means of reducing the risk of exposure. To quote Carlos:

We are told [by the mass media] to use condoms, that famous athletes are infected . . . and about prevention campaigns. All these things gradually make you learn.

In short, there was widespread awareness among participants that AIDS is a disease caused by a virus (in some cases explicit mention was made of HIV), that there is no cure, and that it is life threatening. Moreover, most were also aware that sexual intercourse was the principal means of transmission, and that everyone, whether gay, straight, or bisexual, is equally at risk.

It is clear that the young men interviewed knew how to protect themselves. Condoms were cited in this regard, as were monogamy and abstinence. Indeed, one might argue that Alexandro's response is typical of the participants more generally:

AIDS is one of the things that leads me to abstinence, because I'm scared. I'm scared to meet a person who wants to have sex that very night because just as that person is easy with me, she could have been just as easy with anybody else who had AIDS. That's why I won't have a sexual life with someone I don't know real well, that's why I avoid the heat of the moment, I try to handle the situation, so I don't lose control.

In some cases male participants have taken their faith in science's power to protect them from AIDS a step too far. On one hand, this is evident from the views expressed by certain individuals that pills or vaccines are available to counter the spread of STDs, including AIDS. On the other, a number of young men said that they were afraid of becoming infected through kissing or contaminated cutlery, having heard that HIV resides in any and all bodily fluids.

As for masturbation, there was broad consensus among the male participants that it is a harmless, albeit pleasurable, pursuit. Thus, there was little support for the Church's position that it is sinful, with most indicating that the practice is "normal" or "commonplace." Indeed, some went so far as to argue that it is a bodily need. As Carlos put it, "Masturbating is like taking a bath—it's a normal part of everyday life."

Even among the minority who were opposed to masturbation, their reasons were grounded less in religious dogma than in their own sense of logic and reason. Thus, while some argued that "one isn't giving love to anybody," others said that they do not do it because "women were invented to have sex with."

Young men's understanding of homosexuality was similarly cloaked in the trappings of science and reason. Drawing heavily upon psychoanalytical theories of sexual orientation, participants deemed it the product of an "abnormal" childhood or adolescence. Thus, while Santiago suggested that it was the fault of parents who did not give their children the appropriate cues early in life, others, such as Ivan, argued that it stems from having only sisters. In still other cases, alternative explanations were proposed, such as the view that homosexuality could be traced to incidents of rape or sexual abuse as a young child.

Of course, the mere fact that young men in Villa del Sol understand sexual orientation to be rooted in environmental rather than genetic factors does not make them any more tolerant of homosexuality in their midst. Indeed, one might go so far as to argue their perspective has made them even more intolerant of gays and lesbians, since they are fearful that homosexuality is "contagious" and that individuals can be "converted" to it. Consider statements by individuals such as Jorge, who said that "Everyone can do as they like, homosexual, heterosexual, whatever, as long as it doesn't affect me or other people."

The issue of virginity elicited a similar response among male research participants. That is, most equated it with a state of mind or particular psychological orientation; by contrast, relatively little emphasis was placed upon the sex act itself. Of course, such a view of virginity has led young men in Villa del Sol to attach greater importance to it than their counterparts in Villa del Mar, where it is only seen as noteworthy in relation to women, since they are thought to be the only ones who undergo a discernible physical change in the wake of their first sexual encounter (i.e., they lose their hymens).

Given this perspective, it is not particularly surprising that male participants in Villa del Sol generally supported the view that men—as well as women—should abstain from sex prior to marriage. In Santiago's words:

> Because there are many venereal diseases, you have to reserve
> yourself for the person you love, because if you don't, later on
> you will feel emotionally discouraged and get very depressed.

However, be this as it may, it is clear that male participants placed
greater stock in women's virginity than their own, with Aaron in
particular stating that, "If a woman has sexual intercourse she's no
longer pure. She must be chaste, less experienced, have higher
moral standards and values." Meanwhile, others suggested that,
even though it is preferable for men to remain celibate until their
wedding night, they are often under strong pressure to have sex, if
only to fulfill the "macho" expectations of the society in which they
live.

Finally, it should be noted that there was a high degree of sensitivity among participants to the fact that they are adolescents, and
that this is the stage in their lives when they are prepared for the
responsibilities of adulthood. To quote Aaron, "This is when you try
new things and gain the experience necessary to be an adult." This
perspective is typical of the vast majority of male participants who
hailed from middle- and upper-class family backgrounds, who saw
their teenage years as a time for study, travel, and enjoyment.

Male Discourses in Villa del Mar

We have already suggested that religion plays a very important
role in the day-to-day lives of Villa del Mar community members.
Lacking access to educational and financial resources, individuals
invoke the power of God as a means of saving them from problems
such as poverty and illness. Greater significance is also attached to
physical strength, since it allows men to defend their interests or to
get one of the few available jobs in the construction or fishing
sectors.

However, this is not to imply that scientific discourses are absent
from Villa del Mar, as young people here are no less exposed to
messages disseminated by the mass media than their counterparts in
Villa del Sol. Still, they are more likely to accept and internalize
those discourses which accord most closely with their own realities
and interests. It is precisely for this reason that Villa del Mar's
young men draw so heavily upon essentialism in accounting for

existing gender roles and relations. They believe that men's superiority is grounded in their physical strength and aggressiveness, just as the domination of women can be justified by women's weakness and submissiveness. As discussed at the beginning of this chapter, a similar understanding pervades these individuals' reading of sexual orientation. Homosexuality is thought to be grounded in one's genes, and manifests itself through an unnatural femininity in the case of gay men, and an unaccountable masculinity in the case of lesbians.

One might argue that the emphasis placed by young men upon the body and physical processes is equally discernible in other aspects of their thinking on sex and sexuality. For example, among those who supported birth control measures, most argued that their importance lay in the fact that they ensured that no family member went hungry. Of course, others rejected family planning methods out of hand, chiefly on religious grounds. As Isidro put it, "The family exists to have children, as many children as possible."

The use of condoms appears to be broadly supported by male participants in Villa del Mar, in theory if not in practice. That is, despite widespread awareness that condoms help prevent unwanted pregnancies and reduce the risk of STD infection, many went on to admit that they often do not use one. Although several reasons were cited for this failure to do so, by far the most common explanation was that it reduced sensitivity, thereby reducing the pleasure associated with the sex act. This perspective lends further credence to our argument that Villa del Mar youth see sex primarily as a physical experience rather than a psychological one.

Still, this is not to suggest that reduced pleasure is the only reason why young males often refrain from wearing a condom. On one hand, many felt that it was up to their female partners to ensure that one was used, since women are the ones who run the risk of becoming pregnant. On the other, several individuals indicated that they found it difficult to gain access to condoms, since there are no large supermarkets in the town, and many smaller stores simply do not stock them.

As for AIDS, although male participants clearly have a basic understanding of its dangers, this awareness is undermined by the fact that many have fallen prey to myths and misinformation concerning the disease. It seemed that participants had little sense that they were personally at risk of contracting the virus, a finding that stands in sharp contrast to Villa del Sol, where several individuals indicated that their fear of AIDS had made them decide to abstain from sex altogether. The relatively unconcerned attitude prevalent in Villa del Mar can be explained by the presence of far more immediate problems in the minds of young people there, among them poverty, crime, and drugs. In the words of several young men whom we interviewed, "Everybody has to die of something."

Participants' understanding of the causes of the disease was generally quite weak. Not only was there little awareness of the link between AIDS and HIV, but few appeared to realize that the disease almost always ends in death. Participants' knowledge of the key modes of transmission was stronger, though even here misconceptions existed, with several individuals suggesting that one could become infected through the exchange of saliva.

Meanwhile, in terms of prevention, condom use was the only method cited. No one could think of alternative strategies that might be used to reduce the risk of infection, including abstinence and masturbation. However, in spite of this, participants did show themselves to be sensitive to the fact that AIDS is a disease that can strike anyone, regardless of sexual orientation. As Mainor put it:

> I think that at this time, everybody's at risk, because before it was thought that this was mostly a homosexual and lesbian disease, but I think that we should all be better informed so as not to suffer what other people are suffering.

Turning to the question of masturbation, it is obvious that this is a far more contentious issue in Villa del Mar than it is in Villa del Sol. Although several participants did express support for the practice, for reasons similar to those identified by their middle-class counterparts (i.e., it is a biological "need"), many were strongly opposed, having assimilated religious views on the matter. Yet, even in these cases, it should be noted that the decision not to masturbate is made less because it is a sinful or wicked pastime than because of fears of subsequent punishment. Thus, whereas Louis and Lenin believe that the practice brings about physical or mental illness, Mainor suggested that others can tell when he has been masturbating:

> People talk . . . friends and adults see you on the street and tell
> you, "You've been jerking off, haven't you? You better stop
> because you know it's bad for you." Maybe they're just kid-
> ding, but I think they're right in a way.

Along similar lines, it is clear that young men have assimilated the
Church's position on premarital celibacy as well, particularly for
women. However, as with other issues, stress is laid upon the physical dimensions of virginity, with the presence or absence of a hymen being the key determinant of one's status. Of course, many go
on to argue that, since men have no hymen to lose, virginity is
simply not an issue for them, a perspective espoused by Lenin in
our interview with him: "A man can do anything he wants, but a
woman, she's the one you'd like to get a virgin."

Finally, with regard to participants' understanding of adolescence, the vast majority adopted a strict chronological definition,
suggesting that it is the period roughly between the ages of twelve
and eighteen. In other words, unlike those in Villa del Sol, there was
little emphasis upon such pursuits as "study" and "enjoyment."
Rather, attention was focused more or less exclusively upon
changes taking place in the body, with several young men citing
puberty, growth of body hair, and a deepening voice as key indica-
tors of adolescence.

Female Discourses in Villa del Sol

From our interviews with young men in Villa del Sol, it was
evident that they perceived scientific and religious discourses to be
diametrically opposed. Although this perspective was also evident
among the young women who participated in the study, it was less
pronounced, and there was a general unwillingness to accept "scientific" principles that call into question the sanctity of marriage or
heterosexual relationships more generally.

Thus, it is not especially surprising that female participants were
familiar with key family planning methods, and all were in favor of
their use. Reasons for their support ranged from the need to look
after one's body to fears regarding the economic costs of a large
family. Moreover, it should be noted as well that the young women
had little difficulty in reconciling their position on family planning

with adherence to the Christian faith. As Tatiana put it, "The Church is not going to support me or my children." In any case, most were clearly of the opinion that economic considerations outweighed all others, as the following statements make clear:

> You can't have children just like that. There are poor people who have five or ten kids and they don't have the means to support them. Then they should have only one or two, or only as many as they can afford. (Ileana)

> I think I do support family planning because it's no good to have a lot of kids all in a row and anyway a woman's body gets tired. You have to see people's economic status to see how many children they can afford to have. Family planning is pretty important for everybody. (Maria)

Meanwhile, with regard to condoms in particular, female participants were aware that they are useful both in preventing pregnancy and in reducing the risk of STD infection, and all had a clear understanding of how to use them, regardless of whether they had had their first sexual experience or not. Gianina is typical:

> Well, let's say this is the penis [shows her finger]. You take the condom, you put it here [points to the upper part of her finger], you pull it down, and at the end there's some space with air so that the semen stays there.

Moreover, there was also broad consensus among the young women interviewed that condom use is vital for protection from AIDS and other dangerous diseases:

> I use condoms because I can't say I know my partner real well—you never know who you're with. He can look real healthy, but you never know. So I just protect myself. (Nadia)

> It prevents venereal disease and pregnancies and I know it's not a hundred percent safe, but it's safer than a lot of other gadgets around, it's the safest method there is, you don't muck up your body. (Paula)

However, despite this seemingly favorable attitude toward condom use, it is clear that many participants find them a nuisance at best, and repulsive at worse. For example, several made note of their profound embarrassment at having to walk into a store and buy them. In the words of Alexandra, "You should have seen how embarrassing it was. We went to the cashier and he just stared at us. I don't know, I think the man should buy them, not the woman." Others' discomfort was even more strongly felt, with a number of participants commenting upon the degree to which they were repelled by them. To quote Sophia:

> There are classmates of mine who use them of course, but there are others who buy them just to show off . . . and it's disgusting. Well, at least to me condoms are disgusting, they're so soft-like. My girlfriends also think they're totally disgusting.

This statement serves to underscore the fact that young women in Villa del Sol have greater difficulty in coming to terms with the use of condoms than their male counterparts, a finding that has clear implications for AIDS-prevention initiatives among this segment of the population.

Still, there can be little doubt that female participants are aware of the dangers posed by HIV/AIDS, with most of the young women agreeing that it is a venereal disease, transmitted through sexual intercourse and contaminated blood, and that it has no cure. Condoms were identified as the principal means of prevention; other prevention strategies, such as abstinence, were not mentioned.

Significantly, and in sharp contrast to the young men of Villa del Sol, female participants had little faith in science and its ability to protect individuals from HIV and AIDS. For example, several young women expressed skepticism at experts' claims that one cannot become infected through kissing, while others noted that they were fearful whenever they received an injection. However, by the same token, all of the participants agreed that everyone is at risk, regardless of age or sexual orientation. Drawing once again upon Sofia's words:

> Everybody's at risk, because, you see, a baby can be born like that, or you could have a transfusion with contaminated blood,

or teenagers through sexual intercourse, adults too, or a little boy can be raped. So everybody's at risk.

As for masturbation, the young women who took part in the study were divided as to whether it was a sinful pastime or not. Among those who were opposed to it, most felt either that it made no sense, or that it was an affront to God. Supporters, by contrast, suggested that it was a natural, normal activity, with Adriana in particular arguing that "It's part of growing up, when teenagers start to experiment with their bodies."

With regard to homosexuality, female participants were generally in strong agreement with their male counterparts that its causes are environmental rather than genetic. Thus, while some blamed it on the lack of a male role model in the home, others, such as Priscilla, suggested that it was the product of "too much pampering or ill-treatment." However, this is not to suggest that all of the young women felt this way, with two exceptions being Gisella and Maria, who argued that gay men and lesbians are "born that way, it's in the genes, it's hormonal."

Regardless of their position on the roots of homosexuality, there was relatively little concern among female participants that they might become "tainted" through contact with a gay or lesbian individual. Needless to say, this view sets them apart from the young men of Villa del Sol, among whom fears of "infection" are widespread.

Virginity is another issue that sets Villa del Sol's young women and men apart. While many suggested that the ideal relationship was one in which both partners remained celibate until marriage, it was widely felt that it should be up to each individual woman to decide what course of action is best for her. In the words of two participants:

> I think that's how virginity is: a woman who is virgin is pure and a woman who is not is just as good, just as special, just as intelligent. If she's not virgin it doesn't matter, it's one more experience. (Paula)

> A woman who wants to remain virgin is virgin, and a woman who doesn't is not; it's a personal decision. (Gisella)

These responses underscore the degree to which feminist values and principles have been internalized by young women living in Villa del Sol. That is, not only do they believe that there should be equality among the sexes, but they are particularly resentful of the hypocrisy and double standards inherent within macho culture. Consider the following statements by female research participants:

> I just don't understand—why should a woman be expected to remain chaste until marriage but not a man? (Sophia)

> They can go around having sexual relations with girls and all, so why don't girls also have the right to have sex? If later they marry a woman who's not a virgin, that shouldn't matter. (Paula)

> It's not fair, because just as a man has the right to have sex with a woman, a woman should have the right to have sex with a man. This doesn't mean the woman is a prostitute or something. (Gisella)

Finally, with respect to female participants' understanding of the concept of adolescence, it seems that there are both similarities to and differences from the views expressed by their male counterparts. On one hand, there is general agreement that it is, in essence, a transitional period between one's carefree existence as a child and the burdens of adulthood. As Gisella put it:

> For me, adolescence is the time when a person has to stop being a child and start being an adult and exercising responsibilities, because when you're a child you practically have no responsibilities, but when you become an adult, then you have to set goals for yourself and decide what you're going to do in life.

On the other hand, many also saw it as a stage when their freedom of action began to be circumscribed by the watchful eyes of their parents and families. Thus, several participants commented upon the fact that they were no longer allowed to go out by themselves, or were forbidden to associate with boys. Of course, this in turn is related to the second area in which male and female perceptions differ. While the former tended to associate the onset of adolescence with a particular age, young women identified it instead with their first menstruation or the onset of breast development.

Female Discourses in Villa del Mar

Given that there are relatively few prospects for socioeconomic advancement in Villa del Mar, it should come as no surprise that young women who live in this community tend to see marriage and a devout life as their best hope for the future. Of course, not only does this mean that cohabitation and motherhood come at an early age for many of the women here, but there is a marked tendency as well to discount or discard any discourse that compromises their chances of establishing a family.

Birth control is a case in point. As the interviews and group sessions made clear, Villa del Mar's young women knew relatively little about the efficacy and types of methods available to them, and few felt that lack of knowledge in this area was especially problematic. Still, it must be acknowledged that family planning does have supporters among those whom we interviewed, with several young women commenting upon their usefulness in limiting the size of one's family. In the words of Dunia, "It's good because, without it, all of a sudden you'll realize you've got a whole lot of kids."

As for the usefulness of condoms in particular, most female participants were aware that they help prevent pregnancy and STD infection. However, despite this level of consciousness, only a minority reported making regular use of them. Why is this the case? On one hand, several participants indicated that it was the man's responsibility to decide whether or not one should be worn, since he is typically the more experienced of the two.

On the other, many thought condoms impracticable because of their supposed impact upon sexual pleasure. As Alexandra put it, "Having sex with a condom isn't the same thing . . . it's better without one." This view supports our argument that young women and men in Villa del Mar attach more importance to physical processes and the body than their counterparts in Villa del Sol. Still, in one respect at least, women from the two communities are similar:

both groups indicated that they felt very embarrassed whenever they went into a store in search of condoms.

With regard to HIV and AIDS, although female participants had a basic understanding of the disease, its dangers, and principal modes of transmission, their level of awareness was not as high as that of young women residing in Villa del Sol. Not only did their reluctance to use condoms lead the women to discount them as a prevention strategy, but most did not see themselves as likely victims in any case. Even in those instances where participants did acknowledge a degree of risk, they generally felt that others, among them prostitutes, *playos*, and men, were in much greater danger of becoming HIV positive.

Interestingly, however, female participants' tendency to associate homosexuality with AIDS does not necessarily mean that they are willing to condemn this segment of the population out of hand. That is, despite widespread adherence to an essentialist understanding of sexual orientation, few felt that individuals should be rejected solely on this basis. In Wendy's words, "I wouldn't spurn them because after all they're human beings."

If Villa del Mar's young women are prepared to tolerate homosexuality among their friends and family, one activity that they are most definitely *not* prepared to tolerate is masturbation. In short, while some argued that masturbation is something that women simply do not do, others attacked it in the harshest possible terms, a position that clearly reflects the Church's own condemnation of the practice.

The Church's influence is also evident in young women's views on premarital sex. Most felt strongly that they should "save" themselves for their future husbands, arguing that a woman's virginity is one of her most valuable assets. As Daisy put it, "Ever since I was a little girl I knew I should remain virgin until marriage, because you're supposed to remain clean, free of sin." Significantly, in spite of the fact that a minority of participants did defend their right to engage in sex outside of marriage, very little criticism was heard concerning men who failed to remain celibate. In explaining this silence, one might point to the relative weakness of feminist ideology in Villa del Mar, along with women's willingness to tolerate sexual double standards for the sake of their relationships with men.

Finally, with regard to young women's understanding of the significance of adolescence, most expressed an opinion similar to that of their male counterparts in Villa del Mar, and associated it with a particular chronological period in their lives, stretching from the onset of puberty to their late teen years. Although a small number of participants did make reference to the opportunities that adolescence affords for dances, trips, and the like, most did not see it as a particularly special time in their lives. Indeed, some went so far as to say that their adolescent years were even less enjoyable than those which had preceded them, given that they were now faced with all manner of restrictions on their movements and activities.

Chapter 9

Learning and Imposition of Discourses

It need hardly be emphasized that discourses have neither agency nor the capacity to reproduce themselves. Although it is true that they are vigorously promoted by the groups that derive greatest benefit from their existence, they also depend upon the active collusion of society members in general, who reinforce and sustain them through any number of discursive practices. For example, patriarchal gender discourses are reproduced through practices as diverse as the tendency to elect far more men to Congress than women (equally true for Costa Rica and the United States) and parents' tacit encouragement of aggressive behavior among their male children.

However, even if the benefits associated with a given discourse are not spread evenly across all segments of society, their expanse is usually wide enough to ensure that most people prefer to sustain the status quo rather than risk engaging in practices that might undermine it. Still, the complexity of the social fabric is such that no discourse is able to command absolute hegemony, providing individuals with an opportunity to disregard, reject, or reinterpret specific elements without calling into question the entire discursive edifice.

As for questions related to sexuality in particular, young people assimilate dominant mores and values through a feedback mechanism in which a dualistic worldview produces polarized sexualities that serve in turn to promote and reinforce the internalization of dualistic sexual discourses. In this way, young people's capacity to operate within a compartmentalized sexual culture turns crucially upon their successful adoption of an internal control system that arranges, controls, and censures contradictory information.

TRANSMISSION OF MESSAGES

In Foucault's estimation, power is wielded rather than possessed, necessitating forms of analysis that are focused less on institutions themselves than on the means by which the latter are capable of producing "docile bodies" that are amenable to discipline and control (Foucault, 1978). Sexual discourses are one of the key fields of knowledge through which this is accomplished, and thus it is our purpose in this chapter to explore how they become "anchored" in young people's minds.

Of course, in embarking upon this project, we do not wish to suggest that institutions such as the Church, state, or mass media are somehow unimportant. Indeed, given the resources they command, they are anything but irrelevant in the dissemination of messages about sexuality. For example, churches play a key role in the lives of community members, especially in Villa del Mar, where they distribute food and clothing to the poorest families and organize social, cultural, and educational activities for young people. Similarly, universities are able to shape individuals' views and outlook by virtue of their monopoly over the distribution of diplomas and degrees. Those who wish to become accredited as "professionals" in their field must prove themselves willing to operate within the bounds of the dominant paradigm; otherwise they risk mediocre grades at best, and expulsion at worst.

This point is crucial, revealing as it does the multifaceted nature of disciplinary power. While one might argue that coercive force is the ultimate sanction imposed upon those who fail to conform, other methods are no less effective. These include the threat of job loss for workers who refuse to become complicit in their supervisor's sexism, or girls' fear that they will be thrown out of their home should their parents discover that they are sexually active.

However, it should be noted that, in most cases, these threats need never be carried out, since individuals learn from an early age to accept the tenets of dominant discourses and adapt their behavior to them. As one might imagine, the preeminent site for the imposition of such discourses is the home, where mother, father, siblings, and the extended family all play a part in the inculcation of appropriate values and norms.

Thus, with respect to religion in particular, it is generally the mother or grandmother who teaches the child basic principles and requires him or her to attend Mass, catechism classes, and other church-sponsored activities. This was confirmed in the group and interview sessions, where young people such as Maria and Aaron indicated that they went to church principally because of parental pressure. Although a number of participants went on to describe their fear of being denied intimacy by family members should they fail to live up to the latter's expectations, by the same token it is clear that many also used religious devotion as a means of building power alliances with particular relatives, or of attacking those who did not live up to community expectations in matters of faith. To cite but one example, Isidro reported to us that he has continued to attend Mass regularly in the two years since his mother left his abusive father for another man, despite the fact that she no longer goes to church regularly herself. In short, he saw this as a way of publicizing his disapproval of his mother's "immoral" conduct.

Along somewhat similar lines, several female participants referred to the distinction between "good" and "bad" girls, with the former enjoying a measure of moral superiority over the latter. Needless to say, public demonstration of one's faith plays an important role in this regard, with sexual promiscuity closely associated with an irreligious outlook. Thus, while Anna believes that her personal devotion places her in the camp of those who enjoy an unsullied reputation, she is well aware that there is another group of "misguided and headstrong" girls in her community who have failed to develop a fear of God.

As for gender-centered discourses, the observations of project ethnographers show quite clearly that both mothers and fathers are involved in the teaching process. On one hand, male siblings are forced to compete for their father's approval by acting in a sufficiently masculine fashion, for example by being successful in sports or having many girlfriends. On the other, mothers are also complicit in the reproduction of a patriarchal gender order, to the extent that they teach their daughters to be submissive while expecting their sons to be domineering and aggressive. Although many women engage in such practices simply because they have themselves come to accept patriarchal relations of power as "normal," others do so in order to protect their daughters from what they perceive to be the dangers inherent in a man's world.

LEARNING AND REPETITION

Although young people internalize hegemonic discourses in a number of ways, including most notably blind acceptance, dissemination of essentialist or dualist precepts, and repetition, the last is by far the most common. For example, in the Roman Catholic Church, the same interdictions are touched upon by the priest in almost every Mass, with both Hilda and Santiago commenting upon the repetitive nature of the sermons and how bored they feel each time they go to church. Similarly, Maria, who goes to a denominational school run by nuns, indicated that she is exposed to religious exhortations and prayers more or less constantly.

As one might imagine, repetition is also important in ensuring that individuals behave in a manner that is "appropriate" to their gender. Thus, while girls are continuously reminded of the dangers of going out alone or after dark, boys are similarly pestered if they do *not* wish to go out, since masculinity demands that they be independent, self-reliant, and streetwise.

If by some chance parents are not teaching their offspring appropriate gender behavior, other institutions, among them the mass media, advertisers, the educational system, and the Church, are only too willing to make up for this deficit by offering children and adolescents constant reinforcement as to what is and is not acceptable.

BLIND ACCEPTANCE, ESSENTIALIST THINKING, AND MANICHAEISM

Blind acceptance is another important means through which young people are taught not to challenge or question the status quo. If individuals are to become good Christians, they must show themselves able and willing to rein in their common sense and accept the tenets of the Church on the basis of faith alone. Once they have done so in matters of religion, it becomes increasingly easy for them to suspend their critical faculties in other areas as well, such as human relationships and biology.

Of course, the question of essentialism is highly relevant in this regard, since it is yet another area in which a divine plan or mandate is invoked to explain the Church's position on any number of issues, from women's supposed weakness in the face of temptation to the requirement that priests abstain from all sexual activity. Again, once individuals have learned to accept precepts such as these without question, they are far more likely to assimilate other forms of essentialist thinking as well, for example, in matters of gender role differentiation or sexual orientation. Significantly, this understanding was confirmed in our in-depth interviews with young people, with the latter proving entirely unwilling to challenge essentialist perspectives on a wide range of issues, including those mentioned here.

Along similar lines, the Church is also involved in fostering a Manichaeist worldview among its followers. While this is not to suggest that it is alone in doing so—after all, the modern age is to a large extent founded upon dualistic thinking—its influence is particularly pervasive. At the pulpit and in the Bible, human beings are divided into any number of categories: good and evil, men and women, believers and infidels, saved and sinners. As one might imagine, this emphasis upon dichotomies serves to encourage fragmentation of the personality at an individual level, while lending credibility to the binary oppositions inherent within other hegemonic discourses.

PROSELYTISM

Without wishing to downplay the importance of the assimilation techniques described above, the Church has a near-constant need for recruitment campaigns designed to attract new followers. In both of the communities under study, project ethnographers identified several individuals who devote themselves, on a more or less full-time basis, to the task of convincing others of the verity and power of dominant discourses.

Church officials stand out as particularly prominent in this regard, with priests, parishioners, and young people themselves called upon to convince others of the importance of attending Mass or participating in Church-sponsored activities. However, as active as the Roman Catholic hierarchy may be in attempting to disseminate its message among the Costa Rican population, its efforts pale alongside those of fundamentalist Protestant churches, which enjoy a well-deserved reputation for mounting aggressive proselytizing campaigns. Indeed, they have even gone so far as to democratize the recruitment process, calling upon all members of the congregation to go door-to-door in a concerted effort to win over new converts.

Although a grassroots approach is also used in the popularization of other discourses, most notably those associated with machismo and a patriarchal gender order, such tactics are a far cry from the professionalism that characterizes most state-run reproductive health campaigns. Typically, these revolve around the mobilization of physicians, nurses, social workers, and volunteers in carefully orchestrated drives to promote and disseminate approved messages on a range of health topics.

SOCIAL INSTRUMENTS OF CONTROL:
PUNISHMENT

Reference has already been made to the coercive tools available to upholders of the status quo should the reinforcement techniques described previously fail to prevent "inappropriate" behavior by young people. In the paragraphs that follow, we will touch upon some of the most common forms of punishment deployed against transgressors, including censorship, seclusion, exile, categorization, and violence.

Censorship

As one might imagine, the capacity to suppress or silence alternative perspectives is a powerful weapon in the armory of dominant social forces, and they do not shrink from using it. For example, frank discussion of topics related to sex and sexuality is strongly discouraged in most homes and schools, thereby giving the Church broad scope to communicate its own perspective to young people without fear that they will be contaminated by "illegitimate" sources of information.

Discouragement takes several forms. With respect to female sexuality in particular, our interviews with young women pointed to the existence of what might be called a conspiracy of silence, in which mothers, aunts, and grandmothers (let alone male relatives) simply refused to discuss any issue related to this topic. Thus, not only did most of the participants receive absolutely no emotional support when they began to menstruate, but many felt so uncomfortable with this development that they postponed telling their mothers for as long as possible.

One might argue that families' reticence to discuss menstruation demonstrates their fear of adolescent female sexuality. Quite simply, mothers (and other relatives) associate their daughters' period with the risk of pregnancy, and hence feel that any discussion of it will only increase the likelihood that they will become sexually active. Interestingly, young men face no such taboo in discussing their own sexuality. Though this is certainly not to suggest that families are more likely to provide their sons with sex education than their daughters, it is generally assumed that boys will learn all they need to know on the street, thereby obviating the need for secrecy.

Of course, it should be emphasized that sex is not the only area in which the effects of censorship manifest themselves. Priests and others in the Church hierarchy (both Catholic and Protestant) routinely give warnings concerning the dangers inherent in entertaining beliefs that run contrary to Christian morality or dogma. Should these threats prove insufficient, Costa Rican law includes antiblasphemy provisions whereby individuals who criticize the personage of Christ could find themselves facing a lengthy prison sentence. Given this state of affairs, it is not particularly surprising that research participants had for the most part come to accept religious censorship as normal, with individuals such as Hilda admitting to feelings of guilt whenever she disparages the Church for its misogyny.

Censorship is also invoked in defense of Costa Rica's dominant reproductive health discourses, with physicians taking it upon themselves to ensure that interventions in this area do not pursue "inappropriate" ends. For example, when the medical establishment first awoke to the danger posed by the AIDS epidemic, by no means did it wish to embark upon a prevention campaign that could be perceived as being tolerant of homosexuality. Thus, when a local nongovernmental organization took it upon itself to fill this gap by working directly with the gay community on issues of awareness and prevention, the Ministry of Health ordered it to cease and desist, on the grounds that it was engaged in activities that fell outside of its jurisdiction.

What does all of this mean for young people themselves? According to Jorge, censorship has prevented him from "imagining alternative ways of doing things." That is, the suppression of alternative perspectives and approaches leaves young people with the sense that there is only one answer to any given problem, and that those who fall outside of the mainstream are not only wrongheaded, but evil.

Seclusion

As project ethnographers discovered, seclusion is a strategy employed in both Villa del Mar and Villa del Sol to control or police young people's behavior. Needless to say, its use is particularly widespread among adolescent girls, whose movements outside of the home are carefully circumscribed to prevent them from falling prey either to boys' advances or to their own sexual urges.

It is also used to punish young people who fail to abide by the tenets of dominant discourses. Thus, "unruly" children are often sent to denominational schools as a way of enforcing strict standards of behavior upon them, since such schools are known for their disciplinarian approach and ability to restrict students' access to the outside world. Among those who do not wish or cannot afford to send their children away to a religious school, other forms of seclusion are used, including physical confinement or relocation to the home of another family member elsewhere in the country. As one might imagine, the most common reasons why young people are subjected to these forms of punishment are "promiscuity" (in the case of young women), and drug or alcohol consumption (for young men).

Exile

However, in those instances where seclusion fails to have its desired effect, nonconformist youth are faced with a battery of increasingly severe forms of punishment. Exile is one such measure, and is deployed as a means of insulating the community from discursive challenges or contradictions.

Among those who are targeted in this way, many are young men or women who have chosen to adopt an openly homosexual lifestyle. In short, they are forced to leave their hometown either to save their family from embarrassment, or as a way of avoiding the prejudice and violence of other community members. Other candidates for exile include women who become involved in the sex trade, or young people of both sexes who refuse to support the terms of the dominant gender order.

Categorization

Should "undesirables" of the sort described in the previous section elect to stay in their home community against the wishes of their fellow citizens, they run the risk of categorization. In many ways a form of internal exile, this punishment is invoked when individuals are designated as deviants, prompting other community members to ostracize and ignore them, lest they wish to be considered deviant themselves. As one might imagine, the most common labels in this regard include prostitute, lesbian, gay, drug addict, atheist, and criminal.

Physical and Mental Violence

Still, despite the undoubted pain and suffering inflicted upon young people by the instruments of control discussed in the preceding paragraphs, physical and mental violence remains the ultimate sanction to be used against those who cannot or will not conform. As our in-depth interviews with young people made clear, beatings are often administered to boys who engage in "feminine" pastimes (such as playing with dolls), just as girls who dare to walk the streets by themselves are in danger of being sexually assaulted or raped. Even in cases where there is no physical violence, "deviant" youth, such as effeminate men or masculine women, are forced to contend with a near-constant stream of taunts and threats, engendering a climate of fear which is highly traumatizing in its own right.

INDIVIDUAL INSTRUMENTS OF CONTROL: THE INTERNAL WATCHDOG

Although reference has already been made to the role of the internal watchdog in creating the conditions necessary for individuals to police themselves, thereby ensuring conformity with the principles of dominant discourses, in this section we explore the workings of this "watchdog" further by means of two examples drawn from the in-depth interviews.

In the first instance, we consider the case of Maikol, who was fourteen years of age when he participated in this study. During the course of our interview with him, he admitted that he used to enjoy playing with dolls and braiding his girlfriends' hair. He would also experiment with makeup, try on earrings, and wear his female siblings' clothes, until one day his mother surprised him in the midst of putting on a dress. Although he was punished for doing so, his enjoyment of "feminine" pastimes was such that it was not long before he was caught once again, prompting his parents to become increasingly forceful in their punishments, beating him and locking him in his room for hours on end.

At the same time, family members also attempted to influence his behavior through more subtle means. For example, his grandmother would often take him on long walks as a way of making him "forget" his inappropriate urges, while his father and mother would constantly tell him that he was "no good," that he would never be with a woman, that he would be ostracized and called a "faggot." As Maikol himself made clear, these lessons eventually began to have an effect upon him:

> My mother would hit me and tell me I shouldn't dress like a girl and that I was getting the wrong ideas in my head, and finally I stopped because they scolded me and gave me advice so that I wouldn't forget.

That these "lessons" were successful in making Maikol "forget" his former identity were only too clear to us when we met with him for an interview. Not only did he express gratitude to his parents for discouraging his "bad habits," but he had adopted the manner and opinions of a typical Costa Rican male, arguing that women were the weaker sex and that they should behave in a suitably feminine fashion.

Meanwhile, Leidy is Maikol's mirror image. As a child, she loved to play football with boys, and would often steal away after dinner to hang out with them in the town square. She soon learned that this was not acceptable behavior. Whenever she asked to go out and play, her mother would tell her to stay away from boys, since they were rough and would likely beat her up. In similar fashion, her aunt would turn away any boy who came to the door asking for her, saying that "Leidy is a girl; she's not allowed to play on the street."

Again, with time, these reinforcement techniques began to have an effect, prompting Leidy to adapt her behavior to societal expectations, and causing her to express thanks for the punishment she received as a child: "My mother was right when she told me that men should stick with men and women with women. That's the way it should be."

Having highlighted the degree to which parental reinforcement is capable of altering young people's behavior patterns, we will now explore in detail the specific mechanisms used to foster self-discipline and conformity.

Observation

As is evident from the previous discussion, children are subjected to constant surveillance, their every action scrutinized by any number of authority figures, including parents, grandparents, teachers, physicians, and priests. Of course, constant scrutiny on the part of others prompts young people to be mindful of their own behavior as well, and any action or characteristic that arouses the interest of observers immediately draws the attention of the child who is being watched.

Children quickly learn that adults are extremely interested in gender-relevant behavior, all the more so if it does not correspond to dominant expectations and stereotypes. For example, when Adriana was a young child, she used to play with toy cars. She indicated that she quickly stopped once she realized that her mother was reacting "oddly" whenever she started to play with them. Other participants reported analogous experiences, with Kenneth describing the anger directed toward him by his mother when she discovered him one day playing "house" with a girl. Alberto was similarly upbraided when one of his parents entered his room to find him pretending to be a nurse. As he put it, "My mother was so mad she hurled herself at me, telling me to take those clothes off, they look awful." As punishment, he was sent to the fields and ordered to cut the grass. Finally, Guillerno indicated that although his mother never told him explicitly that he should refrain from playing "house," she would always endeavor to make sure that he adopted the role of a male character, such as the "father" or "husband."

Needless to say, underlying adults' concern that children behave in a manner "appropriate" to their gender is their fixation upon children's genital anatomy, prompting children to pay attention to bodily attributes (e.g., vagina, penis) that would otherwise arouse little or no interest. For example, Marianela admitted that she was completely ignorant of physical differences between the sexes until they were explained to her in the first grade. In her words, "Before that, I thought all children were the same."

As sexual organs grow and become more mature, adults place increased importance upon the physical separation of boys and girls, with interaction between the sexes becoming ever more carefully circumscribed. For example, Juan remembers being bathed by his mother until he was roughly four years old, at which time she abruptly stopped, without telling him why. Similarly, both Santiago and Carlos indicated that they still recall the day when their parents told them that they must leave the washroom while their sisters were bathing.

Of course, in many ways these developments reflect broader changes in the adult-child relationship as the latter's sexual identity becomes more pronounced. As parents are made aware of the fact that their children are sexual beings (e.g., because of penis or breast growth), certain forms of interaction are rendered taboo and off-limits. Thus, among young males in particular, overt signs of affection by fathers and other male relatives become increasingly rare, with research participants such as Jonathan and Guillerno reporting that, while their fathers used to hug and kiss them, they now never do so.

The emphasis placed by adults upon genital organs also serves to encourage young people to discuss and compare them among themselves, often in ways that foster shame and self-consciousness. For instance, Carlos described occasions when he would get together with friends and they would each take off their trousers to determine who had the largest penis. This caused Carlos no end of embarrassment, since his penis was small and the other boys would make fun of it. As for young women, the principal objects of comparison are the breasts, with Hilda in particular indicating that she has always felt ashamed of them, both on account of the fact that she started to develop at an early age, and because boys would often "make comments and joke about the size of them."

As one might imagine, this point is significant, highlighting as it does the fact that surveillance does not cease when children leave their homes. Indeed, if anything, it becomes more intense as they grow older, with teachers, priests, and other community members taking it upon themselves to observe the behavior of the children under their care, and intervene should there be any evidence of "abnormality."

David's experience is typical in this regard. Because he is somewhat effeminate in appearance and manner, his aunt approached his mother one day when he was still quite young, to tell her that she found his conduct "odd" and that she should really "do something" about it. Others followed in his aunt's footsteps, warning his parents of the dangers of such behavior and advising him on how he might go about changing it. Of course, given this background, it is hardly surprising that David remarked (during the course of our interview with him): "I feel like I'm weird and different, like something that's sick."

Indeed, if adults' scrutiny has any effect at all, it ensures that children exercise self-surveillance in order to curb any affectation or behavior that might arouse the censure of those around them, whether authority figures or members of their own peer group. In this way, the need for coercive force diminishes until it becomes almost superfluous. Not only are individuals socialized to think carefully about the consequences of any action they might undertake, but they are also trained to keep a watchful eye on their friends and colleagues, and remind them if they step out of line. For example, several interview participants reported feeling angry whenever their friends complain about having to go to church, or when they talk among themselves during the service.

Confession

Reference has already been made to the central role played by confession within Catholicism. Quite simply, it offers believers a chance to cleanse themselves of the effects of evil thoughts and actions, but only if they are willing to reveal their sins, admit their guilt, and ask for forgiveness.

Regardless of the degree to which such a mechanism is (or is not) useful in helping one cope with personal difficulties or traumatic experiences, there can be little doubt that it facilitates surveillance and control of the population. On one hand, it encourages individuals to categorize their thoughts and feelings, and hide or repress those that are deemed "improper" whenever they are subject to the gaze of parents, priests, or other authority figures.

On the other hand, by "naturalizing" the confessor-penitent relationship, and by associating it with personal development and catharsis, the stage is set for its progressive encroachment upon other walks of life, until such time that individuals' every thought and action are laid bare to any number of self-declared experts, whether psychologists, social workers, lawyers, or marriage counselors.

Tools and Resources of the Internal Watchdog

Thus, while one might point to several factors that are involved in fostering the internal watchdog within each individual, once in place the watchdog is able to draw upon a wide range of mechanisms to ensure compliance with the tenets of hegemonic discourses.

Few are as significant in this regard as one's memory. That is to say, children quickly learn that, if they are to escape the censure of their parents and community, they must forget or repress "inappropriate" feelings and desires. They are also taught to avoid critical thinking whenever possible, lest they uncover discursive contradictions or expose the arbitrary nature of societal prohibitions and taboos.

A second means by which self-control is exercised is through the association of illegitimate thoughts and activities with natural physiological reactions to unpleasant stimuli. In this way, young people learn to equate "perverse" sex acts, including cunnilingus, masturbation, and anal penetration, with "unclean" bodily processes such as urination and defecation. Thus, any temptation they may feel to experiment sexually is counterbalanced by the fact that these activities are perceived to be "naturally" disgusting.

Similar forces are at work when young people are taught to feel shame in response to the exposure of certain parts of their body, specifically those organs associated with reproduction and sexual pleasure (e.g., the breasts, penis, or rectum). Indeed, one might even go so far as to argue that these feelings of shame extend to anything vaguely related to one's sexuality, including romantic fantasies and sexual language.

Of course, closely related to the shame that many young people feel when they look at their bodies in a mirror or purchase condoms in a neighborhood store is the guilt underlying their relationship with parents and other family members. That is, children, far from being encouraged to see themselves as independent, autonomous human beings, are constantly reminded that they are mere appendages, whose every word and act reflects upon the family that raised them. Needless to say, this in turn forces children to be ever-mindful of their behavior, lest they embarrass their parents or bring their name into disrepute (for example, by becoming pregnant outside of marriage or adopting an openly gay lifestyle).

Chapter 10

Contradictions and Compartmentalization

During the course of this work, it has been our contention that young people do not internalize hegemonic discourses as though their minds were blank slates upon which information can be inscribed at will. Rather, they modify and mediate discourses even as they assimilate them. Often arising from contradictions, these modifications provide adolescents with the necessary space to choose among different norms and practices or, in certain cases, to challenge outright the terms of discursive domination.

This study has identified three *alternative* discourses (i.e., erotic, romantic, and feminist) on which much of young people's resistance is centered. Without wishing to suggest that these necessarily complement one another, they are similar to the extent that they all promote egalitarian, nondualist sexual models. Thus, even though they are open to manipulation by hegemonic forces, their links with "official" discourses are tenuous, and are as likely to undermine them as being co-opted by them.

ORIGINS OF CONTRADICTIONS

As one might imagine, the complexity of the dominant social order is such that it would be difficult, if not impossible, to identify the precise source of contradictions undermining a particular discourse at any given moment in time. However, by the same token we would argue that the following factors must be taken into account if one is come to terms with the dynamic of change discernable in Costa Rica today.

In the first instance, it is clear that economic (under)development does have a role to play in rendering individuals either more or less responsive to the tenets of dominant discourses. Quite simply, if one lives in a marginal community where medical facilities are rustic or nonexistent, it is unlikely that one will be in a position to comply with the principles championed in national reproductive health campaigns.

In a somewhat different vein, discursive contradictions are also generated by broad-based changes in the social fabric. In the case of Costa Rica, these include the influx of large numbers of North Americans, who brought with them evangelical Protestant religions that are becoming increasingly vocal in their attempt to challenge the religious supremacy of the Roman Catholic Church. If this were not enough, hegemonic gender discourses are being challenged by young people who have been exposed to—and internalized—the arguments made by international feminism against continued male dominance.

Finally, there can be little doubt that technological advances also have a part to play in the development of contradictions. For example, the fact that the birth control pill is now available to a wide swath of the country's female population has had far-reaching effects in a number of areas, loosening the grip of patriarchal discourses upon women's lives, while rendering many of the Church's sexual teachings irrelevant and backward.

CONTRADICTIONS AND YOUNG PEOPLE

As our interviews and group sessions with young people made clear, they are well aware of the contradictions inherent in the sexual messages they are subjected to on a day-to-day basis. Even in primary school, their teachers' unwillingness to discuss anything vaguely related to sexuality and reproduction is interpreted by them to mean that the subject is too indecent to be broached, and that adults are simply too uncomfortable to raise it any case.

As children grow older, the contradictions become increasingly stark. Thus, while girls are told to abstain from sex until their wedding night, boys are encouraged to have as many relationships as possible. Whereas both boys and girls are taught to view marriage as the only form of union acceptable in the eyes of God, they look around their community and see many types of relationships coexisting side by side.

Soap operas and fashion magazines are continuously emphasizing the importance of romantic love, making girls and young women feel that they must provide their boyfriends with "proof" of their affection, for example by consenting to sex. However, this in turn is countered by their mothers, who tell them to distrust men, and by the experiences of friends and family members who have been abandoned by their boyfriends as soon as they became pregnant.

In this way, even as young people assimilate contradictory norms such as those described above, they cannot help but compare them to their own realities, in the process realizing that those who demand high standards of behavior from them are often those who are most hypocritical in their own sexual lives and practices.

Villa del Mar

As one might imagine, widespread socioeconomic marginalization in Villa del Mar ensures that the gap between what is demanded of young people in the realm of sex and what is actually possible in light of their circumstances is particularly wide. Thus, at the same time that community members place great stock in the supernatural and the spiritual as means of compensating for their lack of material prosperity, their bodies remain the principal tool through which they seek to obtain recognition and pleasure.

This is an important point, serving to highlight the disjuncture between what is desirable and what is possible within a given social context. In other words, young people in Villa del Mar champion marriage and other Christian values precisely because they offer hope for the future, even if the best they can expect right now is bodily pleasure through whatever means possible.

As an example, consider the life histories of Raquel and Wendy. Ages fourteen and seventeen respectively, both have grown up in poverty-stricken, single-parent households. Both are what might be described as conservative in matters of sex, with Wendy in particular emphasizing the importance of premarital virginity and a relationship model based upon a male breadwinner and a female nurturer who is willing to make sacrifices for the sake of her husband and family. However, in spite of her strong support for Christian mores, she admitted to having sex with several young men during recent years, though she went on to argue that her actions did not matter "because [she] didn't feel a thing."

Raquel was even more forceful in defending the Christian position on sex and sexuality. As she put it, "For a woman to be respected, she has to dress in white when she walks down the aisle. Otherwise, she's nothing but a whore." As she was questioned further on her views and background, contradictions began to emerge. In the first instance, she revealed that her mother currently cohabits with a man who is not her husband, and has done so on two occasions in the past. Then, after stating in the first interview session that she had never had sex, she subsequently conceded that this was untrue. In short, not only did she admit that she had had her first sexual encounter at age eleven, but she indicated as well that she has slept with a number of boys since that time.

Gender Differences

In the personal interviews and focus group sessions, young people's responsiveness to particular sexual discourses differed considerably according to whether they were men or women. Thus, almost all of the participants in Villa del Mar—of both sexes— voiced strong support for Christian mores and values, men were far more likely to interpret those values through the lens of "eroticism" and prevailing gender discourses. Even as they are told that it is important to avoid sex outside the bounds of marriage, male youth are also aware that their reputations will be enhanced if they have many partners and appear knowledgeable in the area of lovemaking strategies and techniques.

By contrast, female participants placed considerably more stock in the tenets of romanticism, using them as a counterweight to that which is demanded of them under the terms of dominant gender and religious discourses. In particular, young women draw upon the concept of romantic love as a basis for imagining something other than the drudgery, violence, and inequity that characterize most of the relationships around them. It also offers them a means of escaping religious prohibitions on extramarital sex, to the degree that it is possible to claim that they were blinded by love, and thus driven to do something that they would never have done under "normal" circumstances.

Of course, this is not to suggest that men are completely immune to the precepts of romantic love themselves. Among those we interviewed, several young men indicated that they had fallen in love, and it was clear that this had prompted them to change some of their views regarding women and personal relationships. Not only did they now draw a distinction between women in general and their beloved, but they also resisted the urge to look upon their girlfriends as though they were merely a trophy or sexual object, while defending them from the gossip and jokes of their male peer group.

Villa del Sol

As one might imagine, the emphasis that young people living in Villa del Mar place upon bodily pleasure is not nearly as strongly marked in Villa del Sol. Material success and academic excellence are within the grasp of the bulk of the town's adolescent population, and thus most have little incentive to engage in physical violence, break the law, or experiment sexually with animals (all of which are common pastimes for Villa del Mar youth).

It should also be noted that young men in Villa del Sol are far less likely to adopt a strongly misogynist perspective. In short, not only are they familiar with the basic tenets of liberal feminism, but they are aware of the potential benefits to be derived from a partner who is educated and in a position to enhance household earning power through a career of her own. Of course, in this regard it is no coincidence that steady employment is far easier to come by in Villa del Sol than it is in Villa del Mar, ensuring that men need not feel threatened by a woman who works outside her home.

Meanwhile, among Villa del Sol's young women, interviews and focus groups served to highlight the fact that they generally had little respect for religious and romantic discourses, which they saw as perpetuating female passivity and exploitation. Instead, they tended to adopt a broadly feminist perspective, in which happiness was associated with a career on one hand and, on the other, a stable marriage founded upon principles of equality and fairness. Needless to say, it was precisely this latter objective that made most female participants shy away from feminism in its more radical incarnations.

DISCURSIVE CONTRADICTIONS
AND TOLERANCE OF HOMOSEXUALITY

Christian doctrine is unequivocal in its condemnation of homo-sexuality, which it lambastes as a repugnant sin and an affront to God. After all, were not Adam and Eve given explicit instructions to be fruitful and multiply? Although members of the religious hierar-chy may be quick to mobilize such arguments as they attempt to convince all who will listen of the evils of homosexuality, a substan-tial proportion of study participants reported having friendships or regular social contact with openly gay individuals. However, as sur-prised as some may be by this finding, it should be noted that not all young people were equally tolerant, with Villa del Mar youth gener-ally being far more open-minded in this regard than their counter-parts in Villa del Sol.

Although we must ask ourselves why this is the case, it is first necessary to address a more fundamental question: has modernity brought in its wake greater or lesser acceptance of gay practice and lifestyles? Certainly, some writers contend that scientific advances, urbanization, and mass education have provided the basis for a more enlightened attitude in this area (Weeks, 1985). However, evidence presented by other scholars, Michel Foucault most notable among them, challenges this view. This group would argue that modernity has, to a significant degree, *created* homosexuality, with the emer-gent discipline of psychiatry taking it upon itself to identify—and stamp out—such "abnormality" in the population (Foucault, 1978). While this is not to suggest that homosexuals were looked upon in a favorable light in the premodern era, as attested by the zeal with which most European regimes executed men accused of sodomy, persecution remained at a minimum because it was a particular set of practices that were proscribed, rather than a sexual identity per se.

Thus, psychiatry's "contribution" was to transform homosexuality into a mental illness in need of medical investigation and interven-tion, thereby justifying any number of highly questionable forms of therapy (ranging from lobotomies to induced vomiting) in the pursuit of a "cure." As one might imagine, it is precisely for this reason that homosexuality has come to be associated with perversion and sick-ness in modern industrial societies, Villa del Sol included. However, as we will endeavor to make clear in the discussion below, young people in Villa del Mar have been raised in a rather different cultural context, one that makes use of a classification system based upon criteria other than "homosexual" and "heterosexual."

Let us consider this claim in further detail. Quite simply, findings derived from ethnographic observation, interviews, and focus groups show that individuals living in Villa del Mar tend to look upon homosexuality as a form of gender inversion, in which men adopt feminine characteristics while women adopt masculine ones. Since sexual orientation is deemed to be grounded in one's genes, there is little attempt to ascribe blame. Instead, individuals who engage in same-sex relationships are categorized in a manner identical to everyone else: according to their relative "activity" or "passivity." In effect, this means that men who are domineering and aggressive—stereotypically masculine characteristics—can engage in sexual contact with other men without being thought of as gay. Indeed, in this regard one might argue that same-sex relationships are seen in the same light as adulterous affairs and bestiality; while all are forbidden by the Church, they are attractive to men because they provide the latter with an opportunity to assert their manliness through the domination of others.

By contrast, Villa del Sol youth are less tolerant of homosexuality precisely because it is associated with an abhorrent and frightening Other. That is to say, it is understood to derive from "abnormalities" in a child's psychological development, resulting in deviant adults whose sexual habits are not only perverse, but capable of entrapping "normal" individuals as well. For this reason, young people in Villa del Sol are reticent to admit that they know someone who is gay, let alone that they are friends with such an individual. Of course, also pertinent in this regard is the fact that homosexuality is seen as a challenge to the established social order, calling into question all that heterosexual society holds dear.

DISCOURSES AND COMPARTMENTALIZATION

Even acknowledging the willingness of some individuals to mount a frontal assault upon the tenets of dominant discourses, for most young people acceptance is preferable to confrontation. Indeed, among those whom we interviewed, very few could conceive of alternative means of organizing gender relations or the sexual division of labor. Instead, most of these individuals have attempted to structure their lives in such a way that they are able to reconcile discursive contradictions, with compartmentalization proving to be one of the principal strategies used in this regard. The adoption of such an approach allows individuals to resolve differences among the various discourses by adjusting their behavior to match the surroundings or circumstances in which they find themselves at any given moment in time.

As an example, let us consider the case of Maria. Born and raised in Villa del Mar, she lives with her mother, stepfather, and stepsister. Her mother works at a restaurant, while her stepfather, who drinks heavily, finds sporadic employment as a fisherman and seller of lottery tickets. Her parents' relationship is highly dysfunctional, characterized by binge drinking, extramarital affairs, and extreme violence on the part of the stepfather toward Maria's mother.

As for Maria herself, while she is constantly admonished by her mother to be careful around boys and to "save" herself for marriage, male classmates never miss an opportunity to make lewd comments and fondle her breasts. If this were not traumatizing enough, Maria's stepfather began to abuse her sexually while her mother was away at work, and raped her when she was only twelve years old. Left bleeding in her bedroom, she was too afraid to seek help because he had threatened to kill her mother should she tell anyone about this incident.

In subsequent years, the fear she felt toward her stepfather made her spend more and more time away from home, either visiting with friends or in the company of a young man who would soon become her boyfriend. They had not been dating long when she consented to have sex with him, despite her strong support for Christian mores and premarital abstinence. When asked about this seeming paradox, she replied:

> I don't really know why I did it. I guess when you fall in love you lose your head and do things to prove your affection. I had such a terrible experience with my stepfather that I wanted to do it on my own with someone I love.

Needless to say, "losing one's head" is central to the compartmentalization process, providing young people with an opportunity to justify acts that run counter to stated beliefs and principles, while preserving the illusion of behavioral consistency. After further probing by the interviewer Maria added, "I've never stopped believing in virginity and fidelity. When I had sex with him, I wasn't myself, it wasn't the normal Maria." Though some uncharitable observers might argue that Maria was simply using love-induced madness as a convenient cover for hypocrisy, in fact there is every reason to believe that she was sincere in her explanation. After all, one of the defining features of compartmentalization is the fact that it is grounded in the subconscious, from which repressed urges and desires are only allowed to escape in response to a particular set of triggering mechanisms, of which unbridled passion and alcohol-induced intoxication are two examples.

However, they are not the only features; time and space are also highly relevant in this regard, as is attested by Luis' experience. In our interview with him, he reported having regular sexual contact with a male study partner while the two were alone in his parents' house: "I've told him we shouldn't do it, that it's wrong, but when he starts to touch me I get so hot I can't stop. He takes advantage of how horny I am." When asked why he continues to schedule the study sessions at a time when his parents are away, he said simply that "this is when the house is least noisy." Obviously, it has not occurred to him that he is himself implicated in the decision to continue having a relationship with his friend, by virtue of the fact that he is choosing the time and place to meet, "forgetting" that it is precisely because his parents are not home that sexual contact is possible.

In this way, Luis' actions reflect both a polarized mental state (i.e., between rationality and irrationality) and, at a more general level, the bifurcation of physical space (and time) into zones of pleasure and abstinence, law and chaos, godliness and licentiousness. Thus, ethnographic observation undertaken in both communities highlighted a stark contrast between locales associated with "official" discourses (e.g., schools, churches, and department stores), and those where forbidden pleasures and pursuits are allowed to manifest themselves openly (e.g., bars, discotheques, beaches, brothels, and pool halls).

One might argue that each of these spaces embodies a particular set of taboos and prohibitions grounded in the compartmentalization process. Most obvious among these are restrictions associated with gender. Whereas men enjoy unlimited access to spaces of pleasure thanks to the continuing dominance of patriarchal discourses, women may only gain ingress in special circumstances (e.g., within the context of holidays or rites of passage), or at the cost of becoming known as promiscuous and "easy." In a similar vein, the movement of sexual minorities (be they gay men, lesbians, transvestites, or sex trade workers) is also restricted, though in opposite fashion. That is, strict limitations are placed upon their access to sites, such as churches and schools, where "normal" standards and mores apply; if they wish to visit these locales, they must either disguise their identity or be willing to face ridicule and abuse.

As one might imagine, several consequences result from this state of affairs. First, it affords hegemonic forces the opportunity to discipline and dominate marginalized groups, such as gay men and women, by "keeping them in their place," whether at home under the watchful eyes of their fathers and brothers, or out of sight in neighborhoods where "decent" (i.e., heterosexual) members of society would not dare venture.

Second, it promotes a lack of reflectivity among young people in their handling of issues pertaining to sex. Among many of the study participants, there was a strongly marked tendency to engage in abrupt behavioral changes depending upon the circumstances and locale in which they found themselves. Thus, as one of the project ethnographers was surprised to discover, young women who were usually shy and demure at home would become sexually aggressive and gregarious while on an outing at the beach. Of course, it need hardly be added that such sudden shifts in attitude and demeanor do not encourage the adoption of safe-sex practices, since to do so would imply that one had not "lost one's head" after all.

Finally, one might argue that the bifurcation of physical space into zones of pleasure and self-denial reflects a similar distinction made between legitimate and illegitimate sexuality. Whereas most young people tend to associate the former with matrimony, procreation, and the home (i.e., private space), the latter is generally seen in far more alluring terms, embodying such qualities as danger, eroticism, and passion. In turn, this means that young people (particularly men), upon marrying and starting families of their own, will continue to believe that sex can only be truly exciting if it is forbidden, prompting them to seek it out regardless of the risk to themselves and their relationships.

Chapter 11

Formal Resistance to Discourses

Given that power exercised through discourses necessarily benefits some groups more than others, acts of resistance are inevitable. For the purposes of this study, we take resistance to refer to any expression, conscious or unconscious, of rejection of one or more principles of a dominant discourse. It should also be noted that resistance can be either formal or informal. Informal resistance, an issue that will be addressed in detail in the following chapter, is by definition inchoate and unfocused, and may involve anything from refusing to go to Mass on a Sunday, to girls who choose to have sexual intercourse prior to marriage. In both cases, the tenets of dominant discourses are being called into question, yet there is no underlying agenda, nor are individuals necessarily even aware that they are engaging in an act of resistance; in many cases, their purpose is merely to assert a measure of independence from their parents.

Formal acts of resistance are more focused, and are often characterized by the mobilization of counterhegemonic discourses as means of confronting and resisting the status quo. Among the research participants, feminism, romanticism, and eroticism featured particularly prominently in this regard, though it should be emphasized that their capacity to effect change is undermined by the contexts from which they emerge. That is, not only do romanticism and eroticism trace their origins to a distant past in which the prevailing discourses were quite different from those of today, but none is broad-based enough to mount an effective challenge against present-day sexual culture in general. However, this is not to suggest that such discourses are entirely without subversive effect, as we will endeavor to show in the discussion that follows.

EROTIC DISCOURSES

As Foucault (1988) makes clear, eroticism's roots lie in pre-Christian pagan societies, particularly classical Greece. For the most part, these cultures did not seek to circumscribe the sexual practices of their citizens in a manner that would be familiar to us today. Rather, in Greece if not elsewhere, concern was focused instead upon means of ensuring that free men did not become excessively hedonistic (Foucault, 1988).

It is in this context that self-control *(enkateia)* was championed. That is to say, even as Greek thinkers recognized (and celebrated) the joys to be derived from such pursuits as eating, drinking, and sex, they called upon individuals to restrict their pleasure-seeking activities to those times and places when "need, moment, and function" were in harmony (Foucault, 1988, Vol. 3:51). In effect, this meant that one should control one's urges in public (need); only engage in sexual activity when one was suitably prepared to do so (moment); and always endeavor to make sure that partners behaved in a manner appropriate to their social status (function). So long as these guidelines were adhered to, no particular act was forbidden; body and pleasure were as one (Dover, 1989; Cantarella, 1992).

However, if these views were representative of mainstream opinion in ancient Greece, by no means is this to suggest that dissent was nonexistent, as attested by the numerous schools of oppositional thought which arose in the latter centuries of the classical era. Without wishing to overstate their effect upon dominant mores and values within Greek society itself, they clearly provided much inspiration for early Christian ascetics, whose views on sex remain influential within Christianity to this day (Bullough, 1976).

Among those who were critical of permissive tendencies within classical Greek culture, few were more profound in their impact than the adherents of Orphism, a religious sect which believed that the body is a prison for the soul, and that the only means of escape is through purification, self-denial, and ritual cleansing. These ideas would subsequently be taken up and elaborated upon by a number of influential thinkers, including Plato, Pythagoras, and Epicurus, all of whom saw sex as a distraction at best and, at worst, as a degrading and shameful act that placed human beings at the same level as beasts. Needless to say, views such as these would provide ample fodder for later ascetic traditions (including those associated with the early Christian Church).

Male Erotic Discourses

Focused upon the body and its pleasures, modern-day eroticism provides a potent counterweight to the deadening impact of dominant sexual mores and values. Although it is essentially a male discourse, typified by such subcultures as those associated with bars, sports clubs, street gangs, and brothels, it does not necessarily exclude women, so long as they are willing to abide by its principles and share in its outlook. Its subversiveness lies in its opposition to "respectable" forms of sexual oppression, which it challenges through the celebration of "deviant" sexualities embodied by the street and those who might be found there, whether prostitutes, adulterers, gay men, lesbians, or transgressors of categories.

Among those whom we interviewed, it is clear that "street" sexuality holds a strong appeal. Aaron recounted an incident in which his friend lost his virginity to a prostitute, and Mainor described in vivid detail a recent visit to a brothel:

> It was some experience. I went with a group of friends and we were all up on the dance floor with the whores. I began to act provocatively and then one of them grabbed my dick. I got so hot that I came right there in her hand, and the best thing was that I didn't have to pay a cent.

Meanwhile, others derive pleasure from simply harassing sex-trade workers and others whom they consider deviant. As Jorge described, young men from Villa del Sol would frequently travel to downtown San José to tease any transvestite they might find there: "They say really dirty stuff to us and we'll answer right back with even filthier things." Although the potential for violence is omnipresent in these exchanges, one might nonetheless argue that the two groups are joined together by a common language of pleasure, a fact alluded to by Jorge during the course of our discussion: "I love to go because we talk dirty to each other, and you won't find vulgarity like that anywhere else."

Certainly, the street appears to offer ample scope for expressions of sexuality that hegemonic forces would condemn as perverted. For example, Carlos indicated that he and his friends would routinely congregate in a vacant lot to masturbate and compare the size of their penises. Maikol described occasions when he would get together with a group of young men to seduce and later have sex with young girls. As he put it, "I feel funny fucking girls that young, but they're into it and everybody's doing it." Meanwhile, others recounted experiences they and their friends have had with animals, with Carlos in particular describing an occasion when his cousin forced the family dog to lick and suck his penis.

Of course, it is not only young men who are engaging in "deviant" forms of sexual contact; as several participants indicated to us, they are well aware of the fact that anyone—even highly respected members of the community—is capable of falling prey to sexual urges. Thus, Frederico told us that he has seen the parish priest on several occasions drinking and carousing with unmarried women, while another participant was surprised to discover a policeman in the midst of an adulterous affair:

> Not that long ago, I was walking by a hotel where they rent out rooms by the hour, and who did I see coming out but the policeman with one of the neighborhood women who goes to my church. I would never have imagined that she would get involved with a young man, especially since he just got married four months ago and already he's trying to get it on the sly.

Still, whatever one's opinion of these incidents, they all exemplify what is perhaps the most salient feature of erotic discourses: their emphasis upon the transgression of conventional sexual mores and values. Thus, within this context there is scope for flexibility and experimentation, even among men who would never willingly self-identify as gay or bisexual. As David, a young homosexual man, made clear:

> You never know what to expect when you go into a room alone. Masculine men will often ask you to stick your finger up their ass, talk dirty to them, or treat them like a dog. I like to

feel like a woman and don't particularly like it when a man grabs my balls and sucks them, but life is full of surprises.

Kenneth has had similar experiences, albeit from a heterosexual perspective:

Women often enjoy being sadistic and biting you. When I'm half drunk I like a woman to do everything to me and for her to take the initiative. Doing the same thing all the time is boring. One woman made me suck her ass and afterward she hit me with her belt.

Implicit within these "erotic" encounters is a restructuring of conventional relations of power, in which male dominance is replaced, at least temporarily, by a somewhat more egalitarian relationship dynamic. Interestingly, this perspective appears to be confirmed when one compares the different words used to represent the body within the context of gender and erotic discourses.

Thus, whereas the former tends to draw upon violent, power-laden imagery in its description of the vagina (hole, slit) and the penis (staff, snake), the latter generally makes use of far more benign metaphors, such as papaya or pumpkin for a woman's vagina, and banana or sausage for a man's penis. In this way, the conventional view of men's and women's sexual anatomy, in which one is expected to dominate and penetrate the other, is replaced by an understanding based upon mutual benefit and pleasure.

Eroticism also calls into question the mainstream belief that sex is dirty and should always be kept hidden away within the confines of the bedroom. Indeed, among those who took part in this study, many reported engaging in practices that run directly counter to mainstream sexual mores, for example through participation in "circle jerks" where several young men get together to masturbate after watching a pornographic film. To quote Carlos:

Once you get a little horny, you start touching it. Soon, all your buddies are ready and willing and then one will start jacking off someone else until everyone's come.

Sharing sexual fantasies with each other is another way in which male participants derive pleasure, with pornographic magazines and videos playing an important role in galvanizing the imagination. Of course, it should be noted that videos are often used for "educational" purposes as well, since it is quite common for young people of both communities to go to parties whose principal purpose is to screen pornographic films. Not only did many participants indicate that it was precisely on occasions such as these that they saw the sex act performed for the first time, but several commented that they continue to watch them to learn new lovemaking techniques.

Female Erotic Discourses

As we have endeavored to highlight in our discussion, male erotic discourses differ from those associated with patriarchy or the Church in that they fault no one, male or female, for engaging in acts from which they derive pleasure. Although some might argue that it is scarcely surprising that men should be the principal proponents of this discourse, since they do not have to worry about becoming pregnant or being gang-raped while walking home in the evening, this is not to suggest that women are necessarily opposed to it. Indeed, as our interviews made clear, female adolescents are if anything more unhappy than boys with the demands placed upon them in matters of sex: that they should "save" themselves for marriage; that they should not venture out of the home unaccompanied; and that they should avoid any activity that lends itself to sexual self-discovery.

Thus, even acknowledging the reticence of female participants to engage openly with erotic discourses during interview and group sessions, their willingness to discuss related topics, such as romantic fantasies, underscored the degree to which they too subscribed to many of the tenets of eroticism.

"Secret" boyfriends are a case in point. For example, Wendoly indicated that she has been involved in such a relationship for more than a year, taking advantage of the fact that her parents work during the day to go over to his house after school. Although they abstained from physical contact for much of this time, they had recently begun to "make out," an experience that left Wendoly feeling feverish and flushed:

> I felt an emptiness, an emptiness in my stomach, as though I had never eaten a thing in my entire life, and my eyes were all

watery. I felt as though I had a fever; my body trembled all over. I don't know why, but I remained very quiet all day long.

Alexandra's case is similar. Forbidden to have a boyfriend because she is (in her mother's estimation) too young, she has gone ahead anyway, avoiding detection by always ensuring that her parents are out when he comes over. She admitted that he is very forward, and will often push her to see how far she is prepared to go. The incident described below is typical:

> Once my mother went dancing and we were left alone with my brother and sister-in-law. Anyway, we were in the living room and decided to turn out the light. We were lying down on the couch, talking about things, teasing and joking, and then, all of a sudden, we started to kiss . . . and soon he was kissing me here and there, and my body was saying yes, but suddenly I started thinking, God forbid, and then I decided that I should turn on the light before this got too far.

Meanwhile, dancing is another example of female participants' engagement with eroticism. In short, not only does it give young women scope to challenge the passive role ascribed to them by machismo and the Church, but it also provides them with an opportunity to engage in a nonhierarchical, body-oriented experience.

Parents are also sensitive to these issues, which is precisely why many forbid their daughters to attend dances, or else insist that they be chaperoned at all times by an older sibling or adult. However, as the interview findings clearly show, young women have adopted a number of strategies to bypass or subvert the restrictions placed upon them. Thus, while Daisy takes advantage of visits to some of her more permissive relatives to go out to nightclubs, others, such as Rosangela, sneak out of the house while their parents are sleeping or otherwise occupied. In all cases, however, participants stressed their love of music and the way that it made them feel good about themselves. To quote Alexandra:

> The music, that's what I love most; any kind of music will do. Not like my mother, who dies when you put on reggae and says that it's dirty and not really music at all. Anyway, I love it

all: salsa, romantic, merengue, everything, and if it's good
dance music, so much the better.

Along somewhat different lines, the interviews and group sessions also showed that young women harbor erotic desires and
fantasies that fly in the face of dominant societal expectations of
what female sexuality should and should not entail. For example,
while several participants indicated that they enjoy nothing more
than watching men walk down the street, others said that they went
to sports matches simply to ogle men's muscular bodies and hairy
legs.

It was clear that many of the female participants had exceedingly
rich fantasy lives, as attested by Daisy's dreams of "making love on
a rainy day with romantic music." Similarly, Hilda indicated that
she often imagines herself having sex in a park or public washroom,
anywhere that she would run the risk of being seen. Of course,
nourishing these fantasies are the stories young women tell each
other about the joys of sex and the attractive men they have seen at
school, on the beach, or in magazines.

Thus, even though women are forced to contend with far greater
pressure than men to avoid any and all sexual contact prior to marriage, many draw upon erotic discourses in their pursuit of alternative means of expressing their sexuality. One such means is "petting," consisting of intense hugging, kissing, and manual stimulation,
which is undertaken with lovers and other male friends "with rights."
Needless to say, the latter group is particularly interesting in this
regard. It includes young men on whom a woman has bestowed the
"right" to make love to her without expecting any commitment in
return.

As one might imagine, it is but a short step from petting to genital
intercourse, and though few of the girls and young women interviewed were willing to discuss this issue explicitly, in many cases
such activity could be inferred from the anecdotes they related
about the experiences of girlfriends and female family members.
For example, Alexandra was quite adamant that all of her friends
had already had sex:

> Of my three best friends, I'm almost sure none of them are
> virgins. You see, two of them went with their boyfriends to

sleep by a river and the other one went on a trip with her boyfriend and didn't come back until the day before yesterday. They lied to their mothers and told them they were going to visit some relatives, but the truth is that they were with their boyfriends. According to them, they didn't do anything, but who's going to believe they slept by the river with their boyfriends and they didn't do anything?

Certainly, many boyfriends are exceedingly insistent in this regard, as this quote suggests:

After a few months, he had asked me so many times to give in, to give him my virginity as proof of my love, that one day [when] we were alone and went to a beach, I felt so much desire, it felt so good to have him touch me all over, that I couldn't resist. Next thing I knew he was penetrating me. Sometimes you have this uncontrollable urge. (Leidy)

Lesbian relationships are another form of erotic transgression that most female participants would not admit to, even if it was obvious that some had prior experience in this area. In particular, a number of young women noted that they had been propositioned or harassed by lesbians in the past, with Dunia stating that on several occasions she has been faced with women who call her "cutie" or "sweetie," and who "flirt openly" with her. In our interview with Hilda, she asserted that "most of [her] friends have had little flings with other girlfriends," and went on to describe an encounter she had had some years previously:

When I was about six years old I had a little thing with the girl next door. We used to kiss and kiss. I had forgotten what we used to do until I talked to a friend at school about it and then I remembered. I think my first attraction was to this girlfriend. I loved her very much and she was my best friend.

ROMANTIC DISCOURSES

For the most part, scholars agree that the notion of romantic love originated in the cultural context of twelfth-century Europe, when stories of errant knights and virtuous, unattainable women first began to circulate among the elites of the day. In these works, love was platonic and rarely consummated, with heroic men undertaking seemingly impossible quests for the sake of their ladies' honor (Johnson, 1983).

Although it has undergone substantial change over the course of intervening centuries, this tradition of romantic love remains with us to this day, and is continuously disseminated through such channels as television soap operas, music, and film. Indeed, as Johnson (1983) makes clear, its power to give meaning to individuals' lives is, if anything, stronger than ever, replacing mysticism as the path to true happiness and sexual sublimation.

Our interview findings show that romantic discourses hold considerable appeal for both men and women. In the case of the latter, these discourses offer a means of resisting and subverting the sexual mores embodied by Christianity and science. Meanwhile, romanticism affords men the possibility of having a relationship that transcends the vulgar objectification typical of mainstream gender discourses. In this way, having idealized the woman he is involved with, a man becomes willing to make sacrifices on her behalf, and shelter her from the barbs, gossip, and insults that men routinely direct toward women whom they consider to be sexually active.

As one might imagine, passion plays a key role in this regard, as it is used to justify and explain behavior that runs counter to personal self-interest, as well as the tenets of dominant discourses. That is, individuals who are in love are expected to devote themselves wholeheartedly to their partners, regardless of the consequences. Indeed, it is precisely on this basis that romantic discourses sanction premarital intercourse and other sexual practices condemned by the Church, presenting them as signs of each partner's undying love for the other.

While one can scarcely describe romanticism as a feminist discourse—after all, many would argue that its emphasis on essentialist identities serves only to reinforce patriarchal sexual roles and relations—one should not discount its significance, particularly in marginal communities such as Villa del Mar. On one hand, it provides women (and men) with a means of resisting those who seek to control and circumscribe their sexuality by forcing them to remain celibate outside of marriage. On the other, it serves as a useful device in explaining why relationships fail, and why the reality of marriage so often does not live up to one's hopes and expectations.

Gender and Class Differences in Romantic Discourses

That romanticism is a discourse that does not hold the same appeal for all social groups is implicit within the previous discussion. Thus, let us now address these differences in a somewhat more explicit fashion. In the first instance, it is obvious that women are generally far stronger proponents of romantic love than their male counterparts. This is the case for several reasons, not least of which is the fact that it offers them a potent alternative to the misogyny that permeates mainstream gender and religious discourses. In other words, women champion romanticism precisely because it embodies the prospect of a personal relationship that is loving and non-hierarchical, rather than one founded upon deceit, domination, and violence.

Of course, the institution of patriarchy ensures that men do not feel the same need or interest to partake of a "romantic" relationship of this sort. Not only do they derive personal benefit from women's subservience in the context of a marriage or common-law union (e.g., through housekeeping, personal, and sexual services), but dominant gender constructions are such that men tend to attach relatively little importance to interpersonal relations in their lives. However, this is not to say that men remain entirely unmoved in the face of romantic discourses. On one hand, many are attracted by the warmth and emotional support inherent within a "romantic" relationship. On the other, the fact that men have already internalized certain tenets of romanticism as part of their upbringing in a macho cultural context (e.g., that they must be willing to fight those who show disrespect for their girlfriends) makes them more likely to look upon it with favor than they otherwise would.

Finally, our research findings show that Villa del Mar youth tend to be considerably more enthusiastic in their support of romantic discourses than their counterparts in Villa del Sol. This is the product of several factors, of which one of the most significant is the dearth of opportunities for socioeconomic advancement in this community. Given this state of affairs, local youth see romanticism as the only viable path toward personal fulfillment, a view that stands in sharp contrast to prevailing opinion in Villa del Sol, where young people place far more emphasis upon such issues as psychological compatibility and potential earning power when choosing a suitable mate.

FEMINIST DISCOURSES

Tracing its roots to nineteenth-century Europe and North America, feminist discourse became increasingly influential in the decades following the end of World War II, when changing social realities prompted a growing number of women to mobilize in an effort to advance their personal, political, and reproductive rights. Although the bulk of this activism continues to be centered in first world countries, other regions have benefited as well, with Costa Rica being a notable example.

Without wishing to engage in gross oversimplification, one might nonetheless argue that, for much of its history, feminist ideology has drawn heavily upon liberal political theory, particularly its concepts of reason and the public-private division. In the first instance, early feminist thinkers such as Mary Wollstonecraft (1792/1989) sought to make use of the liberal notion that individuals enjoy certain inalienable rights founded upon their ability to reason, using it as a basis to challenge the palpable inequality of women and men in the societies in which they lived.

Although this strategy did prove to be successful in a number of important respects, for example in garnering women the right to vote, it was not until the second half of the twentieth century that feminists began to make significant improvements in women's day-to-day lives. This was an era of rapid welfare state expansion into a growing number of areas that previously would have been considered part of the private sphere (and, hence, areas the state could not legitimately penetrate), and feminists followed hard on the heels of state agents. Their purpose, as in the case of their predecessors in the nineteenth century, was to promote reform by pointing out contradictions between the rhetoric of equality and the reality of continued discrimination, using the courts and the political system as means of challenging the status quo and forcing the pace of change.

However, by the 1970s the limitations inherent within this "gradualist" approach became increasingly obvious to a growing number of activists within the feminist camp, prompting some to forsake liberal feminism in favor of more radical theorizations of the roots of male domination. For this group, the liberal view that sexual equality can be achieved through such vehicles as greater political representation, enhanced educational opportunities, and affirmative action in the workplace is essentially flawed, since it fails to take into account the fact that the institutions of society, such as mainstream gender constructions themselves, are permeated by the ideology and practice of patriarchy. Thus, according to the radical perspective, women will only achieve true equality once all patriarchal structures (including marriage and obligatory heterosexuality) are fully dismantled.

Feminist Discourses by Gender and Class

Within a Costa Rican context, there can be little doubt that feminism holds considerable appeal for a broad swath of the country's female population. Thus, we were not surprised to learn that many of the young women whom we interviewed strongly supported key elements within the feminist agenda, including an end to male violence, freedom to pursue an education or a career, full equality before the law, and an end to men's exploitation of their wives and girlfriends.

However, it should be noted that their support did not extend beyond the tenets of liberal feminism; for example, none of the participants was willing to call into question the institution of marriage or basic assumptions regarding women's nurturing role. Why is this the case? Although there are undoubtedly any number of forces at work, it is clear that fear of the unknown and an inability to question existing norms feature prominently among the reasons why the feminism of most young women focuses merely upon the elimination of patriarchy's most offensive elements. Thus, as far as female research participants are concerned, the wholesale restructuring of gender roles and relations is simply not on the agenda. As Hilda put it, "I don't know how the world could be otherwise. I can't even imagine us being different."

As for the young men who were involved in the study, the majority were opposed to the feminist program, while at the same time expressing strong support for the status quo. Again, this is not particularly surprising; since men derive disproportionate benefit from the existing gender order, what stake do they have in changing it? However, by the same token it must be acknowledged that a significant number of male participants were prepared to make an exception for forms of feminist claims-making that might prove advantageous to them, for example in relation to women's right to an education or to a career.

Of course, it need hardly be added that gender is not the only variable at work in influencing participants' views on feminism; individuals' class background is also relevant in this regard. For example, low self-esteem and high rates of male joblessness in Villa del Mar have contributed to a situation in which men feel particularly threatened by the principles of liberal feminism, and thus are likely to condemn them in especially strong terms. In Villa del Sol, by contrast, where men are more upwardly mobile and patriarchal gender discourses tend to be imposed in a less coercive fashion, there appears to be significantly less male resistance to feminist ideology and practice.

Chapter 12

Informal Resistance to Discourses

From the outset, one might usefully recall the socioeconomic characteristics that distinguish Villa del Mar from Villa del Sol. In general, Villa del Mar youth who took part in this study hail from low-income social strata, in which absentee fathers and single, working mothers are the norm. Moreover, in the absence of readily accessible material and intellectual resources, young people become "body-oriented," seeing the body as the primary means through which to express their gender and sexuality.

Meanwhile, the majority of participants from Villa del Sol were characterized by staunchly middle-class family backgrounds, with professional fathers and stay-at-home mothers. Thus, not only do young people here enjoy a carefree material existence, but they also have access to a high-quality education. This in turn leads them to place less emphasis upon innate physical qualities when defining themselves, and more on the acquisition of status symbols, whether money, expensive clothes, or a prestigious job.

As we will endeavor to show in the pages that follow, social class (along with gender) is a key determinant of the forms of resistance adopted by young people at any given moment in space or time.

RESISTANCE BY YOUNG WOMEN IN VILLA DEL MAR

During the course of interviews and group sessions involving female participants from Villa del Mar, we were continuously struck by the young women's seeming inability to communicate opinions, feelings, and abstract ideas, particularly when these touched upon matters of sex. Even among those who had experienced sexual initiation (which typically occurs between the ages of eleven and thirteen for girls living in this community), no one was able to describe the physical differences between men and women, or what distinguishes oral from penetrative sex.

How can we explain this? Although it is true that female youth living in Villa del Mar enjoy limited access to social and educational resources, we would argue that young women's apparent lack of sexual knowledge on a cognitive-critical level is in fact indicative of nonverbal resistance to the tenets of hegemonic discourses. Thus, even though almost all of the female participants launched into their interviews by denying any sexual experience whatsoever, many would subsequently admit to a range of sexual practices, including petting, mutual masturbation, and fellatio. Indeed, some went so far as to admit that they had participated in group sex games and other forms of play in which the loser would be obliged to give sexual favors or watch pornographic films. However, despite these admissions, participants would continue to deny that they were sexually active, since they had not engaged in vaginal intercourse. (This argument would sound familiar in the United States in 1998 when it was none other than the U.S. president who would use it to justify his sexual activities.)

Still, this is not to suggest that young women's resistance to dominant sexual discourses is unidimensional. For example, many are also resentful of the heavy emphasis placed upon biology in sex education classes, along with their teachers' lack of honesty and openness in discussing issues related to human sexuality. As one might imagine, this in turn prompts them to disregard information provided in a school setting, and to make use instead of alternative learning channels, including fashion magazines and television soap operas, which also serve as the basis for romantic fantasies that fly in the face of the demands placed upon them.

Daydreaming is also relevant in this regard, representing a form of resistance whose scope is, in many cases, directly proportional to the degree of repression suffered by individuals at the hands of their parents or other family members. Drawing liberally upon the plots of romantic novels and movies, young women imagine wildly erotic encounters free of guilt and drudgery, along with miraculous solutions to their economic woes and poor employment prospects.

One might argue that involvement in evangelical Protestant churches is another form of resistance for Villa del Mar's young women. Although few could identify with precision what distinguishes the Roman Catholic Church from its Protestant counterparts, it was clear—both from the interviews and through ethnographic observation—that the new churches are especially popular with women.

Why is this the case? First, it is clear that many dislike the misogynous attitude that permeates all aspects of Catholic worship, and thus have turned to Protestantism because it offers greater scope for female involvement in church activities, including its governance structure. Furthermore, young women also appreciate the firm stance on male impropriety adopted by the evangelical churches, seeing it as a powerful counterweight to the double standards inherent within prevailing patriarchical discourses.

Finally, it should be emphasized that, among those whom we interviewed, there was a close correlation between strong opposition to dominant discourses and identification with more masculine roles and behavior. Raquel is a case in point. Having been raised in a family of boys, and allowed to play and experiment alongside them, she has grown up to become a young woman who is fearful of neither decision making nor of openly challenging the restrictions and prohibitions placed upon her as a member of the "weaker" sex.

RESISTANCE BY YOUNG MEN IN VILLA DEL MAR

Like their female counterparts, male adolescents in Villa del Mar have adopted a range of strategies to make manifest their opposition to the tenets of hegemonic discourses. Certainly the most visible of these is the habit many have adopted of wearing their hair long, piercing and tattooing their bodies, and choosing clothes that highlight their muscles and tanned skin. Needless to say, these fashion statements are meant to underscore young men's disdain for Christian notions of modesty and chastity.

Similarly, it is quite common for male adolescents to express their hostility toward the Church and the mainstream values it represents by refusing to go to Mass, or by calling into question the moral integrity of priests and other religious officials. Indeed, young men find few pastimes more entertaining than recounting stories of sexual abuse or impropriety perpetrated by those whom they sarcastically refer to as "God's representatives on earth."

As we will endeavor to show in the following section, young men's strategy of focusing upon priests' hyperactive libidos and sordid sexual encounters stands in marked contrast to the approach favored by their counterparts in Villa del Sol, where it is far more common to use logic as a basis upon which to uncover hypocrisy and contradiction within religious institutions and the individuals who represent them.

Meanwhile, male youth whose fathers have abandoned their families and left their mothers to raise the children single-handedly will often adopt views and opinions that run directly counter to predominant gender discourses. For example, Alberto described his mother as "both the man and woman" as far as household management is concerned, and went on to state that not only is she as strong and capable as any man, but "What's really unfair is the way women get billed as the weaker sex, as though they were made of glass while men are made of iron." For Alberto, individuals who subscribe to such a view are ignorant, as are those who treat their wives as "objects or slaves."

As for matters touching directly upon sex and sexuality, young men in Villa del Mar are no less vocal in their resistance. Thus, with respect to sex education classes in particular, many will show their contempt for the course material by laughing and joking continuously, prompting some female participants to complain to us that the male students made it impossible to deal with the subject in a serious manner.

Of course, it is also common for young men to challenge prevailing sexual mores and values by expressing their sexuality through illegitimate channels, such as premarital intercourse, masturbation, voyeurism, homosexuality, and group sex. Indeed, particularly interesting in this regard is the notion of "friends with rights," in essence an unconventional sexual relationship in which neither party makes a commitment to the other. In this way, by turning mainstream views on dating and marriage on their head, young people engage in a form of group resistance to hegemonic discourses that emphasize purity, fidelity, and virginity.

Also pertinent in this regard is the willingness with which young men transgress place- and time-based taboos on sexual activity, for example, by engaging in intercourse during daylight hours or in public places. For example, Kenneth reported having friends who go to the beach every day after school, armed with binoculars so that they can spy on other young couples (whether hetero- or homosexual) who are in the midst of a discreet sexual encounter.

Along similar lines, several male participants indicated that they went out of their way to befriend members of "deviant" sexual minorities, including female sex trade workers, transvestites, gays, and lesbians. As with other practices that run counter to mainstream community standards, their objective in doing so was to register opposition to sexual mores that circumscribed and limited expressions of their own sexuality.

Finally, one might argue that the numerous young men who indicated to us that they are planning to leave Villa del Mar, either to pursue postsecondary studies or in the hope of finding better-paid work in other cities, are also engaging in a form of resistance, whereby dominant community values are self-consciously rejected or called into question. Thus, rather than aspiring to become "real" men whose masculinity is expressed through physical prowess or domination of others, these individuals are endeavoring to construct an alternative identity, founded upon such pillars as educational attainment or financial prosperity.

RESISTANCE BY YOUNG MEN IN VILLA DEL SOL

In light of the stark socioeconomic differences that distinguish the two communities from each other, it is not particularly surprising that young men living in Villa del Sol do not challenge dominant discourses in the same way as their counterparts in Villa del Mar. Whereas members of the latter group tend to express resistance through their bodies, the former are far more likely to make use of critical thinking as a means of calling into question mainstream assumptions and values.

Indeed, one might even go so far as to suggest that superior reasoning skills play much the same role as strength and virility in Villa del Mar, communicating to others that one is worthy of respect, while at the same time providing the basis for displays of rebellion and resistance.

In many respects, Santiago is typical in this regard, using logic and reason in a bid to counter the seemingly unstoppable forces that have served to turn his life upside down. The son of recently divorced parents, he lives with his mother, who depends on her ex-husband's modest support payments to make ends meet.

Given the acrimonious circumstances that surrounded the break-up, including spousal abuse and sexual infidelity on the part of his father, Santiago is understandably bitter. Not only did he blame his mother for initiating divorce proceedings, but he also began to feel ashamed, dirty, and contemptuous of the Christian God who had, in his eyes, failed him. As a way of underscoring his disenchantment, he turned his back on Christianity, focusing his reading instead upon the scientific writings of Charles Darwin, along with the holy texts of any number of non-Christian religions.

However, at a certain point his criticism of the Roman Catholic Church became so forceful that his mother, father, and teachers began to take notice, punishing him severely for giving voice to such heresies. This in turn prompted him to use "logic" once again in an attempt to resolve this latest crisis, indicating in an interview session that his studies had led him to the realization that "all scientific evidence points to the Christian Bible's unfailing accuracy," and that it was God, rather than the man from whose sperm he derives, who is his true father.

When Aaron was recently faced with his father's death and subsequent community disapproval of his mother for becoming involved with another man, he began to question his own religious beliefs, and decided that the Church must become more "flexible" in its interpretation of the Bible.

Male participants in Villa del Sol also used critical thinking to expose contradictions in other hegemonic discourses, with Guillermo in particular arguing that sexism is both "silly" and "unfair." As he put it, "Why should only women remain virgin before marriage? If the woman has to, the man should do the same." However, by the same token it should be noted that the use of logic in resisting dominant models and assumptions is reserved mostly for individuals who are experiencing significant problems in their lives (such as the divorce of their parents); others are far more likely to use critical thinking on behalf of the status quo, rather than against it.

RESISTANCE BY YOUNG WOMEN IN VILLA DEL SOL

In important respects, Villa del Sol's young women are similar to its young men. That is, they complain of the same communication problems with their parents, and are no less aware of the Church's deep-seated influence in many areas of social life. They also tend to be articulate, expressive, and self-confident, qualities that distinguish them in no uncertain terms from their counterparts in Villa del Mar.

Whereas one might argue that many young women in Villa del Sol challenge the tenets of dominant discourses in a number of significant ways, including most notably the refusal of some to adopt a "feminine" appearance (e.g., short skirt, nail polish, and high heels), others, such as Nidia, have gone further in their resistance. Not only is she willing to proclaim openly that she is an atheist, but her vocal criticism of the elitism, corrupt practices, and misogynous outlook of the Roman Catholic hierarchy is at once damning and eloquent:

> How can you respect the Pope when he carries a diamond-studded cross and proclaims his love of simplicity when he kisses a child in Somalia but doesn't care whether the child has got enough to eat? In addition, why is it that we've never seen a female pope, a black pope, a Latin, Asian, or African pope? They've all been white Europeans, most of them Italian.

Although these charges were serious enough in themselves, Nidia went on to identify other areas in which she believes the Church to be dangerously out of step with present-day realities. In her view, nowhere is this more evident than in the field of women's rights, which continue to be trampled with impunity by a religious hierarchy that appears bent on preserving white male privilege regardless of the cost to anyone else.

Even though she often feels intense shame when she looks at herself in a mirror, she is open with her feelings and frank when discussing her sexuality. This is an important point, for it underscores the degree to which Nidia is attempting to fashion for herself a sexual identity based upon honesty and self-awareness, rather than guilt and self-hatred. Let us hope that more young people follow in Nidia's footsteps.

Chapter 13

Sexual Culture and Barriers to AIDS Prevention

As important as the findings outlined in the previous chapters may be, one question remains largely unanswered: how to the sexual cultures of Costa Rican youth contribute to the spread of HIV/AIDS within the population? We address this issue in detail in this concluding chapter.

CENSORSHIP

Defined as an attempt to hinder the free flow of information as a means either of limiting resistance to dominant discourses or of preventing the emergence of alternative ones, censorship is clearly one of the key barriers to an effective AIDS-prevention strategy in Costa Rica. The Roman Catholic Church, in association with particular elements within the media and public at large, has spearheaded a concerted attempt to censor material dealing with premarital sex and AIDS-related topics by staunchly opposing any moves to include them in the sex education curricula of the public school system. However, while this censoring may prevent an attack on dominant sexual values and mores, it also silences debate on alternatives open to young people who are sexually active or who have questions concerning their sexuality.

This attempt to stifle potential resistance to the dominant religious paradigm has not been extended to the romantic or gendered constructions of sexuality. Rather, the popularity (and availability) of romantic novels, films, and pornography has if anything increased, perhaps because these discourses do not pose a threat to dominant modes of thought, as the messages they disseminate serve to reinforce the religious understanding of sexuality.

Nonetheless, for as long as the dominant ideology remains un-questioned, and sex education remains unavailable, young people will continue to fall prey to unwanted pregnancies and HIV infection in this country. As it stands, they are internalizing a set of values which lead them to believe that active penetration is superior to passive penetration, and that God does not punish good Christians. Of course, once such views have been assimilated, one can hardly expect adolescents to be in a position to make the choices that will allow them to lead healthy, fulfilling sexual lives.

INTERNAL WATCHDOG

Discipline is another means of silencing resistance and contradictions. Through this process, young people learn to police their own behavior, and thus do not have to rely on external forces to keep them "in line." In this way, whenever individuals engage in an activity that, upon reflection, falls beyond the bounds of respectability, their "internal watchdog" is invoked, inducing feelings of guilt and suppressing memories of the offending act. Examples of such behavior include childhood sexual games, along with instances of homosexual contact with friends and companions.

However, forgetting is not the only mechanism young people employ to protect themselves from the consequences of sexual transgression. Denial is also used, most notably by *cacheros* who have sexual relations with other men yet do not consider themselves gay. Of course, among the consequences of these "internal watchdog" mechanisms is the tendency to downplay (or deny altogether) the risks associated with unsafe sex and, at a more general level, to fail to learn from one's sexual experiences. All too often, young people, having "discovered" sexual urges within themselves, attempt to satiate these desires without having the slightest consciousness of AIDS-prevention strategies or family planning methods.

Thus, instead of giving youth the tools with which to take responsibility for their actions, hegemonic forces attempt to control their bodies through fear, guilt, disgust, and shame. In this way, the Church, by condemning all expressions of sexuality that are not directly related to procreation, has made young people ashamed of their sex organs, and caused them to feel disgust at any "illegitimate" sexual act, be it masturbation, cunnilingus, petting, or kissing. As the interviews and group sessions have shown, this shame is also felt when individuals go to the store to buy condoms and other birth control devices. As one might imagine, this is largely because such products are associated with either homosexual or nonprocreative sex, thereby invoking guilt and fear of punishment among the young people involved.

MAGIC-RELIGIOUS THOUGHT

In many cases, the proponents of hegemonic discourses attempt to erase contradictions by demanding that individuals engage in blind acceptance, in other words that they accept discursive premises on the basis of faith alone. Mary's immaculate conception and Christ's resurrection provide obvious instances of Christianity's magic-religious orientation. In effect, these attitudes invoke supernatural explanations for natural events, "resolving" contradictions and tensions by placing them outside of the human realm and in that of magic-religious thought.

Although every society has been influenced to some extent by its magic-religious belief system, in Costa Rica this discourse is still overwhelmingly dominant despite the existence of substantial antagonism and contradiction vis-à-vis other discourses. Consider the fact that Costa Ricans, particularly fundamentalists, widely assume that supernatural forces influence most facets of their lives. Even those who are not devout share these views, and thus it should come as no surprise that many young people believe that gods and devils are intimately involved in their decisions to have intercourse, engage in sexual violence, use condoms, watch pornography, or have multiple partners.

Of course, in adhering to such a belief system, individuals are absolved of personal responsibility for their actions. When a "mistake" is made or the bounds of "legitimate" behavior transgressed, the perpetrator can excuse himself or herself by arguing that a supernatural being had influenced, or even made, the decision to act in a particular way. Thus, if a person has sex while in love, he or she can claim that the hand of a god lay behind this action, and thus explanations need not be sought. Similarly, in the event of rape or sexual abuse, individuals will often attempt to justify their actions by claiming that they had been swayed by the devil. Although this is not to suggest that there is no room for autonomous decision making, young people quickly learn that this is neither the only nor necessarily the best way to justify oneself.

With respect to personal relationships in particular, adolescents have internalized the belief that "scientific thinking" is inappropriate for people who are in love, lest they be considered unromantic or insincere. In this way, young people are often convinced by the argument that partners should be chosen on the basis of physical attraction alone (i.e., Cupid's arrow), and not because of intellectual or personal compatibility. Such a perspective does not lend itself to frank discussion concerning the causes of AIDS and prevention strategies, since sexual intercourse is perceived to be a "magical" space of gods and demons untouched by rational thought or common sense.

COMPARTMENTALIZATION

Young people also attempt to address conflicts and discrepancies in sexual discourses through a process of compartmentalization. Rather than rejecting contradictory behaviors and values out of hand, they are placed in separate mental categories, where they coexist in segregation from one another. In this way, behavior becomes dependent upon the company or situation in which one finds oneself, with individuals losing awareness of the contradictory nature of their actions.

In Costa Rican society, the roots of compartmentalization are threefold: religion, family, and historical background. In the first instance, religion encourages such behavior by demanding unswerving obedience to its precepts, leaving no space for the articulation of alternative positions or perspectives. Unorthodox ways of thinking or acting are silenced to avoid the risk of condemnation or punishment. Second, the structure of the Costa Rican family also reinforces compartmentalization through the central role it plays in young people's lives. In short, not only is it assumed that youth will live at home until they are married, but also that they will rely on their parents to find gainful employment. Thus, loyalty to family values is considered vital, and young people are expected to live for their families as well as themselves. Finally, the country's historical legacy is such that it was relegated to the periphery of the Spanish empire, which meant that social control mechanisms were relatively lax, leaving people free to engage in actions (e.g., sex outside of marriage) that would not have been tolerated in the larger colonial centers of Mexico or Peru.

Because of this, the population has learned to live with stark contrasts between the norms expected of them on one hand, and the reality of their day-to-day lives on the other. Costa Ricans' sexual practices confirm this view. For example, in 1995 more than 40 percent of all births took place outside of wedlock, thereby revealing monogamous marriage to be losing ground and under the threat of becoming a "museum piece" (Madrigal, 1992).

As the number and intensity of contradictory ideas increase, so too does compartmentalization. Costa Ricans have inherited two antagonistic and opposing currents of thought, namely machismo and asceticism. On one hand, they have been taught that sex is a means for men to demonstrate their manliness and, on the other, a cardinal sin. However, these different spheres of life are "disconnected" from each other by compartmentalization. That is, within each person the boundaries between different ideas, beliefs, and behavior become reified, resulting in a situation whereby the "religious" sphere is disconnected from "scientific" thought; the emotional sphere is disconnected from reason (since love and reason are deemed incompatible); sexuality is separated from religion (as the latter is seen as entirely hostile toward the former); and finally, among men in particular, gender is removed from the romantic realm (since men must reject machismo's contempt for women if they are to establish a loving relationship with one).

Given this situation, it is not surprising that young people's sexual culture is also compartmentalized. Even as their parents talk to them about the importance of virginity and fidelity, they look around them and see a world rife with adultery and sexual precociousness. Religious dictates are championed yet often go unfulfilled. To cope with these apparent dichotomies, adolescents have divided their environment in ways that correspond to their own mental categories. For example, bars are seen as spaces where desire and sexuality can be openly expressed. Church, meanwhile, is a place for pious behavior, just as school is for studiousness and rational thought.

In this way, young people's compartmentalized communities correspond to their compartmentalized minds, engendering what are often radical changes in personality as they move from one locale to another. Thus, young women who are reserved and passive in Church may very well become assertive and aggressive when they are at the beach with friends. Similarly, young men who are models of good behavior at home become gang leaders or sexual predators when on the street.

That negative consequences should arise from this dichotomization of space and behavior should be obvious. In matters of AIDS awareness in particular, young people are unlikely to benefit from education and prevention initiatives if they do not perceive a link between the context in which they receive the information (e.g., school or Church) and the context where it could actually prove useful (e.g., in a brothel or at a party).

SEXUAL VIOLENCE

The social construction of gender has profound implications for the nature of social relations among men and women, with violence being merely one of the ways in which individuals (usually men) cope with latent tensions and contradictions within the discourse. In particular, it is used to prevent or punish behavior that calls into question patriarchal relations of power.

For Costa Rican youth, violence has become a means of controlling and asserting ownership over women's bodies. The means through which this control is exercised vary, though in many case the violence is extreme. For example, the day after we conducted an interview with one young woman, she was raped by her boyfriend. As the school's guidance counselor made clear to us in meetings afterward, instances of rape and nonconsensual sex are all too common among the female student body.

Not only was rape reported, but so too was sexual abuse and incest, with one participant in particular admitting to having been raped and assaulted by her own father. Others stated that they had suffered a similar fate. Meanwhile, several of the young men who took part in the study indicated that they often used intimidation, deceit, and alcohol as ways of coercing a woman into having sex with them. When these acts of sexual violence are considered alongside the physical violence that young women experience at the hands of their fathers, brothers, and boyfriends, it should come as no surprise that most have learned to manipulate their bodies and desires in ways that are pleasing to men (for example through makeup or tight-fitting clothes).

In the face of this oppression, women often display symptoms of post-traumatic stress disorder, a learned hopelessness that makes them incapable of responding to new crises. Thus, women may become progressively more vulnerable to male aggression because of the extent to which previous trauma has eroded their capacity to halt abuse.

However, despite the level of violence, it should be noted that the gender system imposes certain costs upon its beneficiaries as well. For example, the association of alcohol with masculinity causes young men to drink excessively, indeed so much so that one community leader in Villa del Mar commented that the community's men have become "submale," given the degree to which machismo has made drunkenness and the dole a way of life. This self-destructive orientation is also apparent in men's tendency to spurn bodily care or preventive health measures for fear of appearing effeminate and weak. Of course, it need hardly be added that a culture which treats half its population as objects and the other half as conquering giants will have difficulty in promoting ideas around AIDS awareness and prevention.

ECONOMIC VIOLENCE

Although Costa Rica's dominant discourses purport to be democratic, offering everyone equal access to their bounty so long as they adhere to certain fundamental principles, in fact they reflect the narrow interests of the country's upper and middle classes. However, despite this inequity in the distribution of resources, members of marginalized communities such as Villa del Mar have been co-opted into accepting the tenets of hegemonic discourses, and in many cases have even become their most staunch defenders.

On one hand, many of the individuals whose lives have been torn apart by the effects of joblessness, violence, substance abuse, and family breakup have been drawn to the redemptive power of Christianity. Thus, whether or not the Church is actually able to deliver on all of its promises, at least it offers the possibility of salvation, something which is very appealing to those who are faced with so many problems. However, as we have argued previously, not only is the Church leadership opposed to birth control and premarital sex, but it has resisted strongly any attempts to discuss these issues in a serious manner.

On the other hand, gender discourses have also been influential in this regard, particularly in poor communities where they are learned and reinforced on the street. That is, not only are women given fewer opportunities by their parents to become self-sufficient (e.g., in terms of education or a vocation), but the dominant gender system is such that their earning power is far less than that of men in any case. Of course, these obstacles contribute in turn to a situation in which women lack the resources to empower themselves, and thus have little choice but to engage in activities that serve to perpetuate the existing gender order.

ESCAPISM

Escapism is yet another means by which young people attempt to deal with the proliferation of conflicting discourses. Substance abuse, music, and dancing are all examples of activities that could become addictive. However, not only do they risk becoming addictive, but many are cofactors in HIV infections as well.

Although young people might abuse drugs or alcohol for many reasons, a number of issues stand out as particularly significant in this regard. In the first instance, they provide a useful means of overcoming inhibitions, allowing men to express emotions normally considered "feminine," and women to become more aggressive and assertive. (A finding noted by the project ethnographer following visits to the countryside outside of Villa del Mar. He witnessed how different and assertive and sexually open these young women were outside the community.) Of course, drugs and alcohol also offer young people a way of escaping from problems of everyday life, whether these involve contradictory messages sent to them by their parents, the effects of divorce, or grinding physical and sexual abuse.

*   *   *

In Costa Rica, *coexistence behavior* has taken on a number of different forms in its hidden resistance to sexual discourses, in the process contributing to the difficulties inherent in AIDS-prevention work among the country's adolescent population. Manifesting itself in censorship, internal watchdog mechanisms, magical-religious thought, compartmentalization, sexual and economic violence, and escape mechanisms, this type of behavior seeks to redress contradictions among the dominant discourses, yet in the end only provides temporary solutions to long-term problems.

If AIDS-prevention programs are to be effective, adequate accounts must be taken both of differences in sexual culture, and the role of gender and class in producing such differences. Inasmuch as each subpopulation responds in a distinct manner to particular events and conditions, it is unrealistic to expect a universal prevention campaign to be effective. Instead, each community should have its own prevention program, with an explicit attempt to represent majorities and minorities, conformists, and dissidents.

Bibliography

Abrahams Vargas, M. (1993). Impacto de los mensajes sobre salud reproductiva transmitidos por radio y televisión en los adolescentes de los centros educativos Metodista y José Joaquín Vargas Calvo. Unpublished dissertation: Universidad de Costa Rica.

Acuña, V. (1978). Historia económica del tabaco en Costa Rica. Época colonial, *Anuario de Estudios Centroamericanos*, 4, pp. 279-392.

ADC (Asociación Demográfica Costarricense) (1986). *Encuesta nacional de fecundidad y salud.* San José: The Demographic Association.

Alarcón Mondrus, M. (1993). Conciencia moral e identidad del yo: Clases sociales. Una propuesta teórico-metodológica. Unpublished dissertation: Universidad de Costa Rica.

Almanaque Mundial (1999). Mexico D.F.: Editorial Televisa S.A. de C.V.

Alpízar Jiménez, J. and Denini Langella, V. (1993). Intentos de suicidio: Análisis de aspectos sociodemográficos, psicosociales y familiares de adolescentes consultantes del Hospital Calderón Guardia. Unpublished dissertation: Universidad de Costa Rica.

Amador Tenorio, N. (1987). Formación y capacitación de comités de promotores de salud del adolescente con énfasis en prevención primaria. Unpublished dissertation: Universidad de Costa Rica.

Arias Araya, M. et al. (1986). Estudio sobre la conducta desviada de los adolescentes y guia para su prevención. Unpublished dissertation: Universidad de Costa Rica.

Barth Vargas, L. (1988). Los jóvenes y la educación para la sexualidad. Unpublished dissertation: Universidad Nacional Autónoma.

Berrón, L. (Ed.) (1995). *Feminismo en Costa Rica?* San José: Editorial Mujeres.

Blanco, R. (1967). *Historia eclesiástica de Costa Rica. Del descubrimiento a la erección de la diócesis.* San José: Editorial Costa Rica.

Brenes, I. (1994). Actitudes y prácticas del aborto inducido en Costa Rica. Unpublished dissertation. San José: Universidad de Costa Rica.

Brenes Varela, G. (1991). Erotismo y moral sexual del costarricense: Un estudio exploratorio acerca de algunas manifestaciones sexuales, eróticas y algunos valores sexuales asociados, en una muestra de trescientos adultos de ambos sexos, cuyas edades oscilan entre los veinte y los cuarenta años, residentes en el Cantón Central de San José. Unpublished dissertation. San José: Universidad de Costa Rica.

Broverman, I.K., Broverman, D.M., Clarkson, F.E., Rosenkrantz, P.S., and Vogel, S.R. (1981). Sex role stereotype and clinical judgments of mental health. *Women and mental health.* New York: Basic Books.

Brownmiller, S. (1976). *Against our will: Men, women and rape.* New York: Bantam.

Bullough, V. (1976). *Sexual variance in society and history.* Chicago: The University of Chicago Press.

Cantarella, E. (1992). *Bisexuality in the ancient world.* New Haven, CT: Yale University Press.

Cardoso, C. and Pérez, H. (1977). *Centroamérica y la economía occidental (1520-1930).* San José: Editorial de la Universidad de Costa Rica.

Carvajal, S. and Carvajal, R. (1979). *Evolución del programa de planificación familiar en Costa Rica: Sétimo seminario nacional de demografia.* San José: Asociación Demográfica Costarricense.

CCSS (Caja Costarricense de Seguro Social) (1994). *Encuesta nacional de salud reproductiva 1993: Fecundidad y formación de la familia.* San José: The Bureau.

CELADE (1988). *Costa Rica: Estimación y proyecciones de población 1950-2025.* San José: Centro Latinoamericano de Demografia.

Chacón Sáenz, M. (1981). Experiencia de grupo operativo con adolescentes de décimo año de un colegio público del Área Metropolitana. Unpublished dissertation: Universidad de Costa Rica.

Chacón Zúñiga, C. (1986). Factores que influyen en el proceso de conformación de la identidad sexual durante la adolescencia: Estudio realizado en un grupo de jóvenes del Liceo de San José. Unpublished dissertation: Universidad de Costa Rica.

Conferencia Episcopal Uruguaya (1992). *Catecismo de la iglesia Católica.* Montevideo, Uruguay: LUMEN.

Congregación para la doctrina de la fe (1987). *Carta a los obispos de la iglesia Católica sobre la atención pastoral a las personas homosexuales* (edited by H. Ospina de Fonseca). San José: Ediciones PROMESA.

Cover, J. (1995). Abuso sexual infantil en poblaciones universitarias. Unpublished dissertation: Universidad de Costa Rica.

De Beauvoir, S. (1953). *The second sex.* Translated by H. Parshley. New York: Knopf.

de Brower, D. (Ed.) (1975). *Biblia de Jerusalem,* (Spanish Edition). Bilbao, Spain.

Dirección General de Estadistica y Censos (1994). *Registro de estadisticas vitales, tabulados.* San José: The Directorate.

Dover, K.J. (1989). *Greek homosexuality.* Cambridge, MA: Harvard University Press.

Engels, F. (1970). *The origin of the family, private property and the state.* New York: International.

Firestone, S. (1970). *The dialectic of sex: The case for feminist revolution.* New York: William Morrow.

FLACSO (1995). *Historia general de Centroamérica.* Madrid, Spain: FLACSO.

Foucault, M. (1977). *Discipline and punish: The birth of the prison.* London: Hazell Watson & Viney.

————— (1978). *The history of sexuality,* Vol. 1, *An Introduction.* Translated by Robert Hurley. New York: Pantheon.

————— (1983a). Afterword: The subject and power, in M. Dreyfus and P. Robinow (Eds.), *Michel Foucault: Beyond structuralism and hermeneutics* (Second edition). Chicago: Chicago University Press.

————— (1983b). *The history of sexuality,* Vol. 2, *The Use of Pleasure.* Translated by Robert Hurley. New York: Pantheon.

————— (1988). *The history of sexuality,* Vol. 3, *The Care of the Self.* Translated by Robert Hurley. New York: Pantheon.

Freud, S. (1917). Introductory readings in psychoanalysis. In *Complete Works,* Vol. VI. Madrid, Spain: Biblioteca Nueva, p. 2319.

Friedan, B. (1963). *The feminine mystique,* New York: Norton.

Gagnon, J. (1977). *Human sexualities.* Glenview, IL: Scott, Foresman & Co.

González, I. (1988). Perfil situacional del joven en el área urbana: Aspectos sociológicos y psicológicos. Unpublished dissertation: Universidad Nacional Autónoma.

Hall, C. (1982). *El café y el desarrollo histórico geográfico de Costa Rica.* San José: Editorial Costa Rica.

Hernández, A. (1985). Análisis sociológico, económico y familiar de la menor infractora en Costa Rica: Años 1976-1980. Unpublished dissertation: Universidad Nacional Autónoma.

Hondoy, M. (1987). Análisis del la reproducción de la fuerza de trabajo de las familias del caserío de San Luis, Chacarita, provincia de Puntarenas (1980-1985). Unpublished dissertation: Universidad de Costa Rica.

Izazola, José Antonio (Ed.) (1998). *Situación epidemiológica y económica del SIDA en América Latina y el Caribe.* Mexico: Fundación Mexicana para la Salud.

Jiménez, G., Lizano, M., and Morales, J. (1982). Un estudio de casos. Características de personalidad del adolescente consumidor de marihuana. Unpublished dissertation. San José: Universidad de Costa Rica.

Johnson, R. (1983). *We: Understanding the psychology of romantic love.* San Francisco: Harper & Row.

Kaschak, E. (1993). *Engendered lives: A new psychology of women's experience.* New York: Basic Books.

Kaschak, E. and Sharratt, S. (1995). Los roles sexuales comparados: Sorpresas en Costa Rica. *Rumbo Centroamericano,* July 11-17.

Kooper Arguedas, G. (1987). Actitudes y prácticas asociadas al autocuidado de la salud, consumo de bebidas alcohólicas y embarazo-maternidad de un grupo de adolescentes de la Unión de Cartago. Unpublished dissertation: Universidad de Costa Rica.

Lagos del Valle, I. (1991). Dinámica social Pentecostal: Un estudio sociológico sobre el crecimiento cuantitativo del pentecostalismo en Honduras. Unpublished dissertation: Universidad de Costa Rica.

Laumann, G. and Laumann, M. (1994). A sociological perspective on sexual action. In *Conceiving sexuality: Approaches in a postmodern world,* R. Parker and J. Gagnon (Eds.). London: Routledge.

Lerner, G. (1990). *The creation of patriarchy.* Barcelona: Editorial Critica.

Madrigal Pana, J. (1989). La esterilización femenina en Costa Rica: 1976-1986, *Perspectivas Internacionales de Planificación Familiar,* Special Edition, pp. 22-27.

———— (1992). *El embarazo no deseado en Costa Rica: Informe de resultados,* San José: ADC.

———— (1994). Esterilización femenina en Costa Rica: Evolución, impacto y determinantes. Unpublished dissertation: Universidad de Costa Rica.

Madrigal, P. and Schifter Sikora, J. (1990). *Primera encuesta nacional sobre SIDA: Informe de resultados.* San José: ADC.

Mahon, M. (1992). *Foucault's Nietzschean genealogy: Truth, power, and the subject.* Boston: State University Press.

Millett, K. (1970). *Sexual politics.* New York: Doubleday.

Molina Jiménez, I. and Palmer, S. (Eds.) (1994). *El paso del cometa: Estado, politica social y culturas populares en Costa Rica.* San José: Editorial Porvenir.

Moreno Moreno, W. (1992). Representaciones sociales del proyecto de vida y elección ocupacional en adolescentes nicoyanos, inscritos y no inscritos en el sistema educativo formal. Unpublished dissertation. San José: Universidad de Costa Rica.

Movimiento Familiar Cristiano (1992). (Pamphlet) Familia rescatemos los valores de nuestra sociedad, Ministerio de Educación Pública, *Semana de Integración Familiar* (twenty-third edition). San José: Editorial ICER.

Ortner, S. (1974). Is female to male as nature is to culture? In *Women, Culture and Society,* M.Z. Rosaldo and L. Lamphere (Eds.). Stanford, CA: Stanford University Press.

Rojas Breedy, A. et al. (1991). Situación actual de la adolescencia en la educación secundaria en Costa Rica y alternativas hacia una salud integral, *Monografías de la Organización Panamericana de la Salud y de la Organización Mundial de la Salud* (91-04).

Rojas Chávez, C. (1992). *Los valores del adolescentes costarricense.* San José, Costa Rica: Patronato Nacional de la Infancia.

Rosero, B. (1979). *La situación demográfica de Costa Rica. Sétimo seminario nacional de demografia.* San José: Asociación Demográfica Costarricense.

Roses, C. (1975). El cacao en la economía colonial de Costa Rica. Siglos XVII y XVIII. Unpublished dissertation: Universidad de Costa Rica.

Rossi, L. and Valsecchi, A. (1980). *Diccionario enciclopédico de teología moral* (Fourth edition). Madrid: Ediciones Paulinas.

Sánchez Rojas, A. (1989). La mujer en la iglesia protestante fundamentalista: Un estudio de casos. Unpublished dissertation: Universidad Nacional Autónoma.

Sawicki, J. (1991). *Disciplining Foucault: Feminism, power and the body.* New York: Chapman and Hall.

Scherfey, M. (1970). *A theory on female sexuality: Sisterhood is powerful.* New York: William Morrow.

Schifter, J. (1985). *La fase oculta de la guerra civil en Costa Rica* (Fourth edition). San José: EDUCA.

———— (1989). *La formación de una contracultura: Homosexualismo y sida en Costa Rica.* San José: Ediciones Guayacán.

Schifter, J. and Madrigal, J. (1992). *Hombres que aman hombres.* San José: Ediciones ILEP-SIDA.

Simon, W. and Gagnon, J. (1984). Sexual scripts, *Society* (November/December): 53-60.

Sosa Jara, D. (1995). *Caracteristicas socio-psicosexuales en la adolescencia: Un estudio en adolescentes de segunda enseñanza.* San José: Asociación Demográfica Costarricense.

Thiel, B. (1977). Monografía sobre la población de la República de Costa Rica en el Siglo XIX, *Revista de Estudios y Estadísticas,* 5, pp. 20-48.

Vance, Carole (Ed.) (1991). *Pleasure and danger: Exploring female sexuality.* New York: New York University Press.

Weeks, J. (1977). *Coming out: Homosexual politics in Britain from the nineteenth century to the present.* London: Quarter.

Weeks, J. (1981). *Sex, politics, and society.* London: Longman.

———— (1985). *Sexuality and its discontents.* New York: Routledge.

Witting, M. (1971). *Les guérrilleres.* New York: Avon.

Wollstonecraft, M.S. (1792/1989). *A vindication of the rights of women.* New York: Prometheus Books.

Index

Page numbers followed by the letter "f" indicate figures; those followed by the letter "t" indicate tables.

Order Your Own Copy of
This Important Book for Your Personal Library!

THE SEXUAL CONSTRUCTION OF LATINO YOUTH
Implications for the Spread of HIV/AIDS

_____ in hardbound at $49.95 (ISBN: 0-7890-0884-X)

_____ in softbound at $19.95 (ISBN: 0-7890-0885-8)

COST OF BOOKS_____

OUTSIDE USA/CANADA/
MEXICO: ADD 20%_____

POSTAGE & HANDLING_____
*(US: $3.00 for first book & $1.25
for each additional book)*
*Outside US: $4.75 for first book
& $1.75 for each additional book)*

SUBTOTAL_____

IN CANADA: ADD 7% GST_____

STATE TAX_____
*(NY, OH & MN residents, please
add appropriate local sales tax)*

FINAL TOTAL_____
*(If paying in Canadian funds,
convert using the current
exchange rate. UNESCO
coupons welcome.)*

Prices in US dollars and subject to change without notice.

☐ **BILL ME LATER:** ($5 service charge will be added)
(Bill-me option is good on US/Canada/Mexico orders only;
not good to jobbers, wholesalers, or subscription agencies.)

☐ Check here if billing address is different from
shipping address and attach purchase order and
billing address information.

Signature_____

☐ **PAYMENT ENCLOSED: $**_____

☐ **PLEASE CHARGE TO MY CREDIT CARD.**

☐ Visa ☐ MasterCard ☐ AmEx ☐ Discover
☐ Diner's Club

Account # _____

Exp. Date _____

Signature _____

NAME _____

INSTITUTION _____

ADDRESS _____

CITY _____

STATE/ZIP _____

COUNTRY _____ COUNTY (NY residents only) _____

TEL _____ FAX _____

E-MAIL_____
May we use your e-mail address for confirmations and other types of information? ☐ Yes ☐ No

Order From Your Local Bookstore or Directly From
The Haworth Press, Inc.
10 Alice Street, Binghamton, New York 13904-1580 • USA
TELEPHONE: 1-800-HAWORTH (1-800-429-6784) / Outside US/Canada: (607) 722-5857
FAX: 1-800-895-0582 / Outside US/Canada: (607) 772-6362
E-mail: getinfo@haworthpressinc.com
PLEASE PHOTOCOPY THIS FORM FOR YOUR PERSONAL USE.

BOF96